Intermittent Fasting 16/8: For Beginners:

How to Lose Weight Quickly and Permanently Without Feeling Frustrated. How to Be Always Motivated in Every Period

Copyright © 2020

All right reserved. No portion of this book may be reproduced, stored in a retrieval system, or transmitted in any form or by any means – electronic, mechanical, recording or otherwise – except for brief quotation in printed reviews without the prior written permission of the publisher or the author.

Table of Contents

Introduction 10

Chapter One 13

  What is Intermittent Fasting? 13

    Methods of Intermittent Fasting 15

    What Happens When You Undertake Intermittent Fasting ... 17

    Answer This Question Before Choosing the Best Intermittent Fasting Method 19

Chapter Two 21

  Myths of Intermittent Fasting 21

    Myth #1: You Are Just Starving Yourself And Wrecking Your Metabolism 22

    Myth #2: You Will Always Be Hangry 22

    Myth #3: Intermittent Fasting Is Nothing But A Fad Diet 23

    Myth #4: It Is Extremely Hard To Stick With Intermittent Fasting 24

    Myth #5: There Are Specific Things You Must Eat When Undergoing Intermittent Fasting 25

    Myth #6: Fasting Never Raises Blood Sugar, So It Is Okay To Take Nuts, Avocados, And Whipped Cream 27

    Myth #8: It Is Extremely Difficult To Get All The Nutrients Or Calories Your Body Needs Within A Short Feeding Window. 30

    Myth #9: Intermittent Fasting Is Nothing But A Glorified Eating Disorder 30

    Myth #10: When You Fast, Your Body Is Deprived Of Vital Nutrients 31

    Myth #11: Intermittent Fasting Causes The Breakdown Of Muscle 32

    Myth #12: Intermittent Fasting Will Make You Hungry

Without Respite, Leading To Overcompensation At The Next Meal 33

Myth #13: Fasting Is Much Better Than Snacking For Losing Weight 34

Myth #14: Breakfast Must Not Be Skipped As It Is The Most Important Meal Of The Day...34

Myth #15: When You Stop Your Intermittent Fast, You Can Eat As Much As You Want..35

Myth #16: It Is Impossible To Work Out When Fasting 36

Myth #17: All Forms Of Intermittent Fasting Are The Same, And Every Person Will Get The Same Results.........................36

Myth #18: You Will Become Extremely Fit And Healthy When You Fast 37

Myth #19: Your Body Never Processes Food At Night, Which Is Why Intermittent Fasting Works.. 38

Myth #20: You Will Lose Weight No Matter What 38

Myth #21: You Should Not Drink Water At All While Fasting 39

Myth #22: Fasting Saps All Your Energy............................... 40

Myth #23: Intermittent Fasting Is For Everyone 41

Myth #24: You Can't Focus While Undertaking A Fast 42

Myth #25: You Cannot Gain Muscle While Fasting 43

Myth #26: There Is A Right Way And A Wrong Way To Engage In Fasting 43

Chapter Three... 46

Intermittent Fasting and the 16/8 Method...............................46

Intermittent Fasting 16/8: What Is It?....................................46

How to Get Started With Intermittent Fasting 16/8 48

Chapter Four 55

How to Be Always Motivated When Undertaking Intermittent Fasting 16/8 55

Set a Short-Term Goal with a Tempting Reward 57

Get a Fasting-Accountability Friend 58

Watch Videos or Read Blog Posts/Articles 59

Close Your Eyes, and Imagine What Your Life Will Look in the Future 60

Recognize What You Need: Sometimes a Stick, At Other Times a Carrot 60

Always Focus on Positive Issues or Things 61

Envision Your Healthy Future 61

Take Note of the Positive Changes You Have Already Experienced 62

Always Be Compassionate or Tender-Hearted with Your Lovely Self 63

Form the Habit of Motivating Yourself 63

Chapter Five 65

The Science Behind Intermittent Fasting 65

Types of Intermittent Fasting 70

What Intermittent Fasting is Not 71

Chapter Six 73

6 Ways Of Undertaking Intermittent Fasting 73

Benefits of Intermittent Fasting 16/8 79

Chapter Seven 91

Drawbacks of Intermittent Fasting 16/8 91

Stress-sensitive people 95

Diabetes 96

Chapter Eight 98
  Benefits of Intermittent Fasting to the Human Brain 98
    Intermittent Fasting Reduces Inflammation 98
    It Creates Even More Brain Cells 100
    It Supercharges Your Energy 102
    Intermittent Fasting Boosts HGH (Human Growth Hormone) 102

Chapter Nine 105
  Fasting and Cancer 105

Chapter Ten 110
  Intermittent Fasting and Your Diet 110
    Choosing the Best Foods for Your Intermittent Fast 111
    Hydration 117
    Exclude these Foods from Intermittent Fasting 119

Chapter Eleven 121
  Is Breakfast the Most Important Meal of the Whole Day? 121
    Combining Specific Diets and Intermittent Fasting 126

Chapter Twelve 130
  Correct Mindset 130

Chapter Thirteen 140
  Intermittent Fasting 16/8 140
    Start Slow 141
    Eat well 141
    Start Hydrated 143
    Avoid Sugary Drinks And Food 144

Minimize Intense Activities 144
Positioning Your Eating Window 145
Signs To Watch Out For 145

Chapter Fourteen **148**
Metabolism and the Thermic Effect of Food 148
Factors Stabilizing Metabolic Rate during Intermittent Fasting
.... 149

Chapter Fifteen..**154**
Strategic Black Coffee during Intermittent Fasting 16/8 154
Profound Benefits of Black Coffee 157
What Else Can You Drink During Intermittent Fasting 16/8?
.... 164
Incorporating Black Coffee in An Intermittent Fasting
Schedule.. 166

Chapter Sixteen **168**
Tips Specific to Intermittent Fasting 16/8............................... 168
Suppressing Hunger During Intermittent Fasting 16/8 168
When to Perform Exercises 169
Skipping Breakfast? 170

Chapter Seventeen **171**
What Are The Four Crucial Healthy Habits Of Life? 171

Chapter Eighteen...**176**
Sleep... 176
Effects of Sleep Deprivation 180
Combating Sleep Deprivation.. 183

Chapter Nineteen **185**
   How to Lose Weight Quickly Without Feeling Frustrated....... 185
      Benefits of Exercise.. 186

Conclusion... **191**

Introduction

Fasting is a very ancient practice that has been in existence for millennia. It plays vital roles in medical and religious literature for almost as long as its existence. To many people, fasting is a way to create that spiritual connection that humanity always seeks, to improve mindfulness, and to find guidance.

The first time you hear the word 'fast,' your mind probably conjures Lent in Orthodox Christianity and Catholicism, meditation fasts in Buddhist schools and Ramadan in Islam. You are not far off the mark.

Traditional Lent usually lasts for 40 days in which one meal is eaten per day while some churches allow more freedom with the fast. Ramadan is a month-long fast in which Muslims don't eat as long as the sun is up and only eat once when the sun goes down. It is, essentially, an 8-12-hour fast with a few hours to eat at night and very early the next morning.

Some Buddhist schools practice fasting to aid in spiritual practices and meditation, which often happens every day. The meal at dinner is usually skipped in such places.

There are several kinds of fasts in spiritual and religious practices. People fast for a wide variety of reasons: for personal, political, and even medical reasons. There was a time when healthcare professionals prescribed fasting for patients who were too ill to eat. The physicians of old believed that fasting would have a tremendous impact on the patient, especially in terms of healing of diseases and injuries.

Although it remains unclear whether such stories were true or not, modern fasting seems to support that analogy. This is because fasting is no longer limited or relegated to religious arenas but openly practiced by anyone who wants to. It is generally associated with improved health and overall wellbeing.

The most popular form of fasting that trends almost every year is intermittent fasting. This fasting involves choosing not to eat for a specified period of hours. For instance, you can fast during the evening and even night hours without snacking during the night. You may even skip breakfast the next day and settle for lunch. Intermittent fasting generally doesn't go beyond a day, which is why you won't find many intermittent fasts over 30 hours or longer.

Intermittent fasting is not starvation and has been proven to be healthy. It offers tremendous benefit to those who want to lose weight or those who want to significantly improve their blood sugar levels or bring down their insulin resistance.

In this book, the basics of intermittent fasting will be covered, including the different types. In particular, intermittent fasting 16/8 will be discussed extensively for beginners, who should try this method of fasting and who should refrain from it. The benefits, risks, and efficacy of intermittent fasting 16/8 and how it is used to combat cancer and other debilitating illness will also be highlighted.

Are you ready to start your intermittent fasting journey and enjoy the benefits it offers? Then join us, and let's begin.

Chapter One

What is Intermittent Fasting?

Intermittent fasting refers to an eating structure or eating plan that cycle between periods of eating and fasting. It is a simple method of scheduling your meals in order to get the best or the most out of them. It doesn't specify the foods you should consume – which is what diet is all about – but focuses more on 'when' you should eat the foods.

There are no special foods to focus on or any food restrictions whatsoever. You won't need to count calories, fats, carbs, fiber content, proteins, micros, macros or any other nutrient. You don't have to purchase any expensive shakes or consume bone broth. This is why it shouldn't be considered as a diet but an eating pattern.

Popular intermittent fasting methods generally involve 16-hour fasts daily or fasting for 24 hours, at least twice per week. Popular or well-accepted eating windows, as they are referred to are 9 am to 5 pm and/or 10 am to 6 pm. You are permitted – within this window – to consume your daily calories.

Fasting is a very ancient practice that has been in existence almost throughout human evolution. Ancient cave dwellers, hunters, and gatherers sometimes went without food to eat for extended periods due to the weather, lack of access to food sources, and so on.

Humans have evolved, and can still function for several hours without food. Fasting occasionally is now even more natural than consuming 3 or 4 meals every day.

Fasting and starvation do not mean the same thing, and what makes fasting different from starvation is control. Fasting is controlled while starvation – which is the uncontrolled absence of food for an extended period – can lead to intense suffering or death. It is not controlled or deliberate.

But fasting, on the other hand, is the conscious avoidance of food or the intake of calories for several reasons. Someone usually does it with enough stored body fat and who is not underweight. Fasting is not meant to cause suffering or death. In this case, food is available, but you decide not to eat it for a specific period, i.e. from a few hours to a few days, with or without medical supervision.

Fasting is also practiced in some religions – e.g. Christianity, Islam, Buddhism, and Judaism – as a spiritual exercise. What many do not know are the benefits that fasting brings to the table if practiced from time to time.

You can begin fasting at will, and you may also end it at any time of your choosing. Any period that you are not eating any food, you are intermittently fasting. For instance, you can fast between dinner and breakfast the following day, which is about 12-14 hours. In that sense, intermittent fasting can be said to be part of everyday life. It is beneficial for heart health, reduces cholesterol, prevents type 2 diabetes, and even lowers blood pressure as well as several other obesity-related conditions, thereby making it a viable option.

Methods of Intermittent Fasting

Intermittent fasting can be done in more than one way; a common thread that runs through them all is that it involves splitting the day or even week into eating and fasting phases. Whenever you are undergoing a fast, you either eat very little or nothing at all.

The following are the most popular methods of intermittent fasting:

- **The 16/8 Method**

This method of intermittent fasting – otherwise known as the Leangains protocol – involves skipping breakfast. And then you may have to restrict your daily eating period to eight hours, e.g. from 1-9 pm.

Then, you will fast for about 16 hours in between. This method of intermittent fasting is the focus of this book and will be discussed in-depth in the coming chapters. In other words, you eat for 8 hours and fast for 16 hours.

Many people who practice intermittent fasting believe the 16/8 method is the most sustainable, easiest, and simplest to stick to.

- **The 5:2 Diet**

This method of intermittent fasting involves the consumption of about 500-600 calories on two uninterrupted days of the week. But on other days of the week, which is up to 5 days, you may eat normally.

- **Eat-Stop-Eat**

This variety of intermittent fast will require you to fast for 24 hours, at least once or twice per week. For instance, you may skip today's dinner and wait to eat dinner the next day.

All these methods of intermittent fasting are geared toward the reduction of calorie intake, which will result in overall weight loss. This is only possible if you do not cheat or compensate by overeating food during your eating periods.

What Happens When You Undertake Intermittent Fasting

When you undertake intermittent fasting – or any fasting for that matter – several reactions happen in your body on both the molecular and cellular level. During that period, your body begins to adjust its hormone levels in order to make stored fat in the body more accessible.

Your cells also start to initiate vital repair processes as well as change all expression of genes. The following are some of the changes that will occur in your body when you start fasting:

- **Cellular Repair**

Human cells engender cellular repair processes during fasting, including autophagy, which is the process in which cells digest themselves and eliminates dysfunctional and old proteins that develop inside cells.

- **Insulin**

Insulin levels drop dramatically as insulin sensitivity improves. The lower the insulin levels, the more accessible stored body fat is.

- **Human Growth Hormone (HGH)**

During a fast, the levels of HGH or growth hormone go up dramatically, and may even increase as much as 5-fold. Increased levels of the human growth hormone facilitate muscle gain and fat loss, to mention just a few benefits.

- **Gene Expression**

Changes in the numerous functions of genes associated with protection against disease and longevity occur.

The numerous changes in hormone levels – which include gene expression and cell function – are fully responsible for the remarkable benefits that come with intermittent fasting.

Answer This Question Before Choosing the Best Intermittent Fasting Method

There are some things that you must consider when it comes to choosing an intermittent fasting method that works for you. If you choose an intermittent fasting method that does not work for you, it will

The whole business of intermittent fasting will only work if you make moves to significantly improve your chances of sticking to the new approach to eating.

Do not force an intermittent fasting method that will not work with your lifestyle and current is an added stress that you don't really need.

This is why you need to provide answers to this question in order to determine which intermittent fasting will work for you and your current situation with diet/food.

If You Have Been Eating Healthy, How Long was It?

The Standard American Diet is sugary and extremely addictive. And intermittent fasting can be very challenging if you are coming right of this high carb diet. If you jump right off into a fasting window, it can trigger sugar withdrawal symptoms that can make it quite difficult to sustain the fast for any considerable amount of time.

This means that how long you have been eating healthy plays a crucial role in your ability to sustain intermittent fasting. This is not to say that you shouldn't undertake the fast if your eating habits is not exactly pristine. In fact, you are a prime candidate for intermittent fasting if you have not been eating healthy.

Chapter Two

Myths of Intermittent Fasting

Intermittent fasting continues to become increasingly popular over the years as both men and women of all races and ages have jumped on the bandwagon of this superlative health and fitness trend to improve their overall health and lose weight. But before you join these wildly enthusiastic individuals on this journey, it is essential for you to clear the air about things that you have heard or read about intermittent fasting that are not true.

There is a lot of skepticism surrounding intermittent fasting, most of which are based on no research whatsoever. Most of the myths exist via misconceptions and assumptions. In this section, the myths surrounding intermittent fasting will be highlighted and debunked as much as possible.

If you are ready, let's take the plunge!

Myth #1: You Are Just Starving Yourself And Wrecking Your Metabolism

Intermittent fasting taps into stored fat in the human body, that is, if you already have stored fat. When you fast, the insulin level in your body plummets, thereby pushing your body out of what is known as 'fat-storage' mode and right into 'fat-burning' mode. This state of the human body is referred to as 'ketosis.'

Now, when your body enters the state of ketosis, it does not affect your metabolism. Your body can tap into the plentiful stores therein in the absence of breath mints, frequent meals, chewing gum, and snacks.

Myth #2: You Will Always Be Hangry

When undergoing intermittent fasting, you will be hangry from time to time. 'Hangry' is a term or adjective defined as hungry and angry, especially when the anger is induced by hunger.

Yes, it is true that you may experience some hanger for a few days, and may even extend to a couple of weeks. But it will eventually go away if you stick with it.

You can minimize early intermittent fasting hanger via slowly building up from regular fasts to longer ones.

Myth #3: Intermittent Fasting Is Nothing But A Fad Diet

As mentioned earlier, intermittent fasting is not a diet in any way, but an approach to eating that involves stopping the intake of calories or food in general for at least 14 hours – or more in some cases – each day. You can eat or drink whatever you feel like consuming afterward. There won't be any food restrictions or eating special meals or foods. You are not mandated to purchase any expensive shakes or force yourself to take bone broth.

You don't even need to count calories, proteins, fiber content, grams of sugar, carbs, or any other nutrient. After the period of fasting, you can cook whatever food you like and enjoy it until you are satisfied. And then you stop eating any food for the day.

Of course, if you want to bother yourself squinting at food labels or counting calories or poring over journals to gauge the morsels that you consume each day, intermittent fasting will not stop you. It is very compatible with your lifestyle, and can only be referred to as a fad by individuals who practice it for a week or two and then quit.

But one thing is clear: intermittent fasting is incredibly effective.

Myth #4: It Is Extremely Hard To Stick With Intermittent Fasting

That is not true. What is truly hard for most individuals who embark on intermittent fasting is keeping away from eating ice cream, enjoying a pizza, drinking a can or two of beer, a taco, or even consuming oatmeal chocolate chip cookies hot right out of the oven.

The exceptional beauty of intermittent fasting is that you can eat anything you want to eat. This means that treats will lose their guilt inducement or gorge appeal since they are not ever off-limits but delayed for just a few hours.

It may even save you some money in the long run as you may eye some goodie or two and promise yourself to enjoy them when your eating window arrives. But you may have forgotten all about it.

The key to sticking with intermittent fasting is not jumping straight up into 24-hour fasts right away. You should start small, at 14 hours at least or even less if you can't bear it. Then work your way up gradually to longer fasts. It will make this seemingly new lifestyle far easier to begin with and stick to.

Myth #5: There Are Specific Things You Must Eat When Undergoing Intermittent Fasting

If you love bone broth, you can always consume it during your eating window. If you also can't live without your diet soda or bulletproof coffee, simply take them during your eating window. Bone broth, coffee, diet soda, celery sticks, etc. have no part in an effective intermittent fast. That means you should stay away from them within the period you are fasting, and this includes nuts, chewing gum, gummy vitamins, etc.

Fasting is fasting; if you want to fast, then fast. The whole point of intermittent fasting is not sticking food into your lovely face all the time.

The only time you have to indulge in your favorite fruit flavored LaCroix, vodka, or anything that floats your boat is during your eating window.

There are clean approaches to fasting in which you can take sparkling or plain water along with decaf or black coffee. In this instance, stay away from fruit-flavored waters or frou-frou flavored coffees. Decaf or Plain black tea is also acceptable; you must not take fruity or sweet herbal teas. The beautiful thing about this particular approach to intermittent fasting is that you will be less hungry than you would be if you stimulated your appetite on your own.

Therefore, do not be taken in by any blogger's or journalist's claim that it is okay to keep stuffing your face while fasting. People want to hear this as no one likes to experience hunger pangs while eating.

But intermittent fasting does not really work that way. The things that you are told it is okay to eat make fasting much harder than it should be.

Myth #6: Fasting Never Raises Blood Sugar, So It Is Okay To Take Nuts, Avocados, And Whipped Cream

Many individuals consume foods that do not really increase blood glucose with those that stimulate insulin production. As long as it is food, insulin will be stimulated. Insulin may also be stimulated if it is flavored sweet. This is why you should not take that chance.

Insulin is one nifty hormone that can switch your body over to fat storage mode in an instant. To burn off fat, you need to cut down insulin production so that your body can readily access and use up those excess fat stores for energy. This is what intermittent fasting does to the human body.

Some foods may not stimulate insulin production, but then your body prefers to take up and burn off the fat in that avocado, a handful of walnuts, or hot buttered coffee before bothering to tap into the stored fat in your body. So, if you are struggling with extreme hunger or losing fat, it is highly recommended that you embark on a clean fast before you consider giving it all up.

Myth #7: When You Stop, You Will Gain Every Weight You've Lost

This may be technically true for nearly every weight loss approach. If you stop intermittent fasting or keto diet, you may start piling on fat again. But the primary reason for putting on weight is because you have gone back to your old eating habits after a few weeks. So, forget about fitting into that new pair of skinny jeans.

It proves one point: all diets work – including intermittent fasting – if you stick to them for the long haul or fail to stop. Moreover, since intermittent fasting is not a diet, as mentioned previously – the advantages it offers are three-fold even after you give it up or stop.

- Intermittent fasting preserves and boosts metabolism. This occurs when your body starts tapping into its numerous fat stores, thereby canceling out the need to slow your metabolism down. This is the same action it undertakes when you consume low-calorie diets. Low calorie-diets stimulate the human body to minimize metabolism in order to match the reduced intake of food. But on intermittent fasting, the human body will not be forced to do that since it can tap right into stored fat.

- As soon as you have experienced the mental clarity and impressive energy of fat-burning mode, you will understand how crappy you have been feeling all these while when you kept stuffing your face with all manner of junks and digesting food all the time. You may end up eating less often even after you are no longer undertaking intermittent fasting.

- Intermittent fasting can correct your appetite so well that your desire for junk food dies off, and you start craving lower quantities of food. Since you only get to eat within a specified period every few hours of each day, you will be pickier while your stomach's overall capacity starts shrinking gradually. So, do not be very surprised if you discover that you no longer have the need or urge to consume fast foods.

Intermittent fasting is a lifestyle; it is flexible, practical, free, and highly sustainable. There is no need to stop intermittent fasting, especially if you feel good about it.

Myth #8: It Is Extremely Difficult To Get All The Nutrients Or Calories Your Body Needs Within A Short Feeding Window

You are not as nutritionally brittle as you probably think. Is it advisable to eat healthy and whole natural foods? Yes, you should; always eat the good stuff and minimize or skip the junk altogether. If you really want to, you can prepare healthy foods the major parts of your diet since you will only need to prepare a meal or two a day when embarking on intermittent fasting.

Fasting can be challenging if you keep stimulating your hunger with snacks, so-called healthy meals or question nutrient profiles, food origins as well as the levels of processing while making up your mind whether you should eat or not.

Myth #9: Intermittent Fasting Is Nothing But A Glorified Eating Disorder

You don't need to be a super rocket scientist to know that you should avoid any approach to food that may trigger you to return to a high-risk obsession. But that is if you have suffered from eating disorders.

Moreover, intermittent fasting is not always the best approach for every individual. People on medications that need to be taken with food or certain health conditions, pregnant women or nursing mothers, and children should abstain from intermittent fasting and look for another recommended approach by health experts.

It is an excellent idea to consult health experts or your doctor before embarking on any major changes in your eating pattern. It must be understood that intermittent fasting is not an eating disorder, but a pattern of eating that alternates brief periods of refraining from eating food with brief periods of regular intake of foods.

You can always focus on other things than food throughout the day and then enjoy a satisfying and healthy meal later.

Myth #10: When You Fast, Your Body Is Deprived Of Vital Nutrients
Long-term research and clinical studies have not revealed any evidence to back up this claim or indicated nutrient deficiency – or malnutrition – in participants that engaged in fasting.

Therefore, what should be emphasized is the quality of the food you consume after breaking your fast. Avoid processed and nutrient-deficient foods as much as possible. Increase the consumption of unprocessed and nutrient-rich foods as these help you to avoid nutritional deficiencies.

And finally, fasting gives the potential for some stored, fat-soluble vitamins to be released from fat stores so that they can be readily accessible. Therefore, fasting does not rob you of essential nutrients in any way.

Myth #11: Intermittent Fasting Causes The Breakdown Of Muscle

Do you know that you may have to fast for 5 or more uninterrupted days before any considerable amount of muscle is employed for energy? Fasting encourages the continuous breaking down and rebuilding of muscle tissue via the promotion of autophagy, which is the clearing away of old proteins to be replaced with a set of new ones.

Studies on intermittent fasting, combined with intense resistance training, have beneficial effects in hypertrophy and strength of worked muscles. This partly occurs as a result of fasting-increased growth hormones.

Myth #12: Intermittent Fasting Will Make You Hungry Without Respite, Leading To Overcompensation At The Next Meal

In-depth studies have shown that when an individual skips a meal, eating slightly more at the next meal is high even though it may not be enough to compensate for that particular skipped meal.

Let's say you eat 500kcals for breakfast and 500kcals at a buffet lunch. If you skip breakfast the following week but still have access to the same buffet lunch, you may end up eating up to 700kcals. As you can see, you have eaten much more than you should at lunch since you skipped breakfast, but overall, it is still less.

Fasting has been proven to significantly reduce the production of hunger hormones that promote appetite while stimulating the production of satiety hormones that foster fullness.

You may feel hungry at first as your body adapts to the new eating style, but you will start experiencing less hunger when establishing an intermittent fasting routine.

Myth #13: Fasting Is Much Better Than Snacking For Losing Weight
When people diet, it is expected that such individuals would snack between each meal. One of the myths of intermittent fasting makes those who try to believe that it is a substitute for healthy snacking.

But the truth is that weight loss boils down to a constant calorie deficit, whether those calories are spread over a full day or consumed within a four-to-eight hour period. Just do your best for your body as well as lifestyle in order to reach preset goals.

Myth #14: Breakfast Must Not Be Skipped As It Is The Most Important Meal Of The Day
This myth is believed even by diehard dieticians, and the rationale behind this is that a big breakfast gives the human body the energy boost it needs to start each day. Cereal companies want you to think that you may not be at your sharpest if you don't eat a big breakfast, which is considered the most important meal of the day.

Suppose you don't take a big breakfast. In that case, your body will compensate for this lack by significantly increasing the levels of growth hormone, cortisol, and adrenaline, which stimulates the liver to produce glucose, thus physiologically giving you the much-needed energy to start your day. This proves that eating food as soon as you wake up in the morning is not all that essential.

The word 'breakfast' is usually linked with eating after waking. Break down the word, and you will have 'break-fast.' As you can see, it does not really matter what time you break your overnight fast.

Myth #15: When You Stop Your Intermittent Fast, You Can Eat As Much As You Want

Intermittent fasting is the start of a healthier lifestyle. But it is unfortunate because many people believe that after fasting, they can always go back to that lifestyle of uncontrolled eating. When you do this, you have basically rubbished all the work that you put in for the intermittent fast, as it will be counterproductive.

The key to being incredibly successful with intermittent fasting is that you should eat as you would typically do when you bring your fast to an end. If you fast throughout the day until dinnertime but proceed to eat a dinner made up of a combined breakfast-lunch-dinner, you have wholly negated all the time you put in while fasting.

Myth #16: It Is Impossible To Work Out When Fasting

According to veteran and certified fitness specialists, it is possible to work out while fasting as it is considered a positive thing.

The best time to engage in exercise is first thing in the morning and on an empty stomach. When you do this, your body quickly starts to burn up the fat already stored in your cells as against the calories from the food you consumed the previous evening. You can eat your breakfast after the workout session in order to replenish your body.

Myth #17: All Forms Of Intermittent Fasting Are The Same, And Every Person Will Get The Same Results

As you well know, there are several forms of intermittent fasting; this means there is no official or authorized definition of what intermittent fasting is. For instance, some intermittent fasting protocols may involve doing time-restricted feeding to a 6,8, or 10-hour window, while others fast daily.

Myth #18: You Will Become Extremely Fit And Healthy When You Fast

The results of intermittent fasting are seen and appreciated when combined with proper care and exercise for weight loss. This is why it must be pointed out that engaging in intermittent fasting alone is not enough or does not guarantee success at becoming fit as a fiddle.

No magic bullet solution exists for losing weight; if you want to enjoy health and fitness, then you must be willing to dedicate some time to maintain them every day throughout your entire life. Never take them for granted in any way.

Yes, fasting will not give you that perfect body overnight, and even if you lose some weight, you should never stop your healthy habits but continue them. This includes regular exercise and a nutritious diet.

Myth #19: Your Body Never Processes Food At Night, Which Is Why Intermittent Fasting Works

One of the major misconceptions about intermittent fasting is that intermittent fasting only works because the human body does not process foods at night. Although it is often said that digestion does not take place after a particular period, this myth is untrue.

The human body digests food, irrespective of what time it is. It is all about giving room for your body – over a specific period – to focus on metabolic processes like cellular repair and autophagy instead of pooling all attention to digestion.

This means that if you eat any food at 3 am, your body will readily digest it.

Myth #20: You Will Lose Weight No Matter What

It may shock you to realize that intermittent fasting – or fasting in general – does not always result in significant weight loss. This is a common misconception that is making the rounds nowadays, according to fitness experts.

It does not matter how long the intermittent fast is for, but you will never achieve your goal of losing weight if you always break the fast by throwing down pizzas, burgers, and even candy. This is an indication that intermittent fast works together with a well-planned healthy diet. As long as you don't treat each fasting period like a cheat day, you will achieve your aim of losing weight.

Myth #21: You Should Not Drink Water At All While Fasting

Some religious fasts, especially Christian fasting, involves restriction from food and water. This may be unrelated to this point or myth, but there are unproven claims that no-water fasts are fantastic and optimal for overall health.

But fasting has a diuretic effect, so restricting the intake of water can result in severe dehydration. This is why health professionals and physicians pay close attention to the intake of fluids whenever they supervise patients that undergo therapeutic fasts. These health professionals also pay close attention to electrolytes such as potassium and sodium, which are part of the constituents peed out during intermittent fasting or any fasting.

Therefore, drink water when undertaking a fast, and for fasts more extended than 13 or 14 hours, you should consider supplementing with sodium and potassium.

Myth #22: Fasting Saps All Your Energy

No one doubts that your energy levels will plummet if you don't take food, which is the human body's fuel. However, when you engage in intermittent fast, your cells turn to and taps an alternate energy source, which is the fat stored up in your body. And there is more than enough fat goes round all the cells in your body.

Even a lean person with just 10 percent of body fat has great fat stores that can support energy needs during a fast. Many individuals who had undergone intermittent fasting report better energy when they performed workouts in fasted states. This makes a lot of sense as blood is summarily diverted away from muscles and the gastrointestinal tracts after large meals.

This indicates that there is no truth to the myth that intermittent fast saps one's energy, which may affect daily productivity.

Myth #23: Intermittent Fasting Is For Everyone

Intermittent fasting is incredibly popular nowadays and is continually marketed as highly beneficial for everyone. But this is far from the truth.

Although fasting is healthy and safe for most individuals, health professionals recommend that some groups of people should steer clear. The group of people that should not attempt intermittent fasting includes:

- Children
- Underweight people
- Pregnant and nursing mothers

These groups of people need as much food as they can consume per day, not less. In reality, the high risk of nutrient deficiency exceeds any potential benefits of intermittent fasting.

Moreover, people with high blood sugar are generally advised to proceed with caution when undertaking intermittent fasting. Fasting may be therapeutic for this particular population; however, medical supervision is a must and highly essential to prevent hypoglycemia or dangerously low blood sugar.

Myth #24: You Can't Focus While Undertaking A Fast

Have you ever been ravenously hungry before? I'm sure it is something that you would never want to experience again. And this is because your cells are not used to such a state for extended periods.

However, adopting a consistent or regular practice of fasting intermittently will not put you in this hangry state as your cells will readily adapt to utilizing body fat for energy as your hunger hormone stabilizes.

Burning up body fat also results in the production of ketones, which are tiny molecules that fuel the human brain with efficient and clean energy. When a state of ketosis is stimulated or promoted, it significantly improves attention, concentration, and focus for seniors.

What you can do for your brain, body, and overall health is simply exceptional when you adopt this flexible eating pattern. Many individuals end up accomplishing much more while fasting, especially after they have been able to get past the numerous misinformed intermittent fasting myths.

Myth #25: You Cannot Gain Muscle While Fasting

At first glance, it doesn't seem as if fasting is an excellent way to build muscle. It is true that the human body needs protein, but not 24/7.

According to a study in 2019, active individuals that practiced intermittent fasting 16/8 gained as much muscle and even strength as those who consumed food on a more traditional routine.

Myth #26: There Is A Right Way And A Wrong Way To Engage In Fasting

Yes and no. People who fast do so for several reasons which include:

- Metabolic healing

- Anti-aging
- Mental and spiritual clarity
- Disease prevention
- Weight loss

To meet every purpose, specific criteria have to be met, or else the fast will not work for that particular goal.

A fast for weight loss, for instance, may allow things that an anti-aging fast wouldn't. When you know why you want to fast, you will also know the particular kind of fast you should adhere to.

One of the most regrettable mistakes today is that many people go on intermittent fasting without finding out more details on how it will help them accomplish their goals. Once this category of individuals read something that doesn't necessarily apply to them, they tend to give up and start feeling like failures.

Some read advice or recommendations for the wrong type of fast and end up doing one or two things wrongly, which ruin all their dedicated efforts.

The human body always works unbelievingly hard to preserve as much muscle as possible during times of perceived scarcity. When you fast, body fat – and not muscles – provides the much-need fuel for energy.

Chapter Three

Intermittent Fasting and the 16/8 Method

As you well know by now, fasting is something that has been practiced for thousands of years across different cultures and religions around the world.

One of the most popular forms or styles of fasting that is prescribed or recommended by social media influencers, Silicon Valley moguls, and celebrities, is 16/8 intermittent fasting. Advocates of this style of fasting – which is also known as the 8-hour diet – claim that it is a convenient, sustainable, and easy way to boost overall health and lose weight.

In this section – and the remaining parts of this book – you will learn what intermittent fasting 16/8 is as well as how it works.

Intermittent Fasting 16/8: What Is It?

Intermittent fasting 16/8 involves limiting the intake of foods as well as calorie-laden beverages in order to set a specific window of 8 hours a day and then abstaining from consuming food for the remaining sixteen hours. Proponents of intermittent fasting 16/8 believe that this approach to food consumption works by supporting the circadian rhythm of the body, i.e. its internal clock or biological time. The primary goal of this time-restricted fasting is to lose weight and achieve better health, though it does much more than that.

This is one cycle that can be repeated as often or as frequently as you like. It may be once per week, twice or even every day, depending on personal preferences. Following this unique method of fasting implies that you will abstain from foods at night and for most parts of the morning the following day. But you can get your daily calories during the day, depending on the schedule that you choose to follow.

The popularity of intermittent fasting 16/8 has skyrocketed in recent years, especially in the circles of individuals looking to burn fat and lose weight. As mentioned earlier in this chapter, intermittent fasting 16/8 is not a diet, and so it is not subject to the strict regulations and rules of diets. However, another school of thought consider intermittent fasting 16/8 a diet plan that is very easy to follow and proven to provide real and measurable outcomes with minimal efforts. It is somewhat flexible and less restrictive than several other diet plans and fits into any lifestyle.

Aside from enhancing weight loss, intermittent fasting 16/8 is also believed to significantly boost brain function, improve blood sugar control, and also increase longevity. Since practically no food is off-limits during the eating window, some enthusiasts tend to supercharge their weight loss by following the keto diet at mealtimes.

How to Get Started With Intermittent Fasting 16/8

Intermittent fasting 16/8 is safe, sustainable, and above all, incredibly simple. Anytime you are not eating, you are intermittent fasting. For instance, if you don't take any solid foods between dinner and breakfast the following day – which spans a period of about 12-14 hours – you have intermittently fasted. This is why intermittent fasting is considered of everyday life in this sense.

However, in order to deliberately get started with intermittent fasting, you should pick out an 8-hour window and then limit the intake of food to only that time frame or span.

Most people that undertake intermittent fasting 16/8 usually prefer to eat between noon and 8 pm. This implies that you may have to fast overnight and then skip breakfast the next day. However, you can eat a well-balanced lunch and dinner. You may also consume a few snacks before the day comes to an end.

Other individuals prefer to eat between 9 am and 5 pm, which gives them more than enough time to consume healthy breakfasts. They can take a regular lunch at noon and a light but early dinner or even snacks by 4 pm before you start fasting. This is what many health experts recommend as finishing food consumption very early in the evening will not rock your circadian rhythm as metabolism generally slow down right after this period. This is, however, not feasible for many people who want to engage in intermittent fasting 16/8.

Another time frame that many people undertaking intermittent fasting 16/8 go for is between 10 am and 6 pm. However, you are at liberty to try a little experiment in order to pick out the perfect time frame that fits your schedule.

Moreover, the best way to fully maximize the health benefits derived from intermittent fasting 16/8, it is highly recommended that you stick to only nutritious whole foods as well as beverages during your eating windows. When you fill up on nutrient-rich foods, you will reap the profound rewards that this approach to eating has to offer.

Always balance each meal that you consume during your eating windows with a wide variety of healthy foods such as:

- **Whole grains**: Rice, quinoa, buckwheat, barley, etc.
- **Veggies**: Leafy greens, broccoli, tomatoes, cauliflower, cucumbers, etc.
- **Healthy fats**: Avocado and coconut oil, olive oil
- **Fruits**: Apples, berries, bananas, peaches, oranges, pears, etc.
- **Protein sources**: Eggs, legumes, poultry, nuts, meat, seeds, fish, etc.

You can also drink water, unsweetened coffee and tea as well as other calorie-free beverages while fasting. This will help you to control your appetite while keeping you well hydrated.

Eating regularly within these time frames is vital in order to prevent excessive hunger, blood sugar dips, and peaks.

You should always shy away from junk food as much as possible so that you don't negate the positive effects linked with intermittent fasting 16/8. It may do your overall health more harm than good. Asides this, there are no restrictions whatsoever on the amounts or types of food that you can eat during the eating window. The flexibility of this plan makes it extremely easy to follow.

Intermittent fasting 16/8 decreases food intake in two different ways:

Decreased Appetite – Many individuals have incomprehensibly reported that they experienced reduced hunger levels while undertaking intermittent fasting 16/8. Decreased hunger levels imply less overall intake of calories, and this leads to greater weight loss.

In addition to this, there may be physiological explanations for decreased hunger from intermittent fasting 16/8. Fasting in general significantly increases ketones which have been proven to bring down ghrelin, the ever-popular 'hunger hormone'.

Decreased ghrelin from intermittent fasting 16/8 could decrease appetite, which will, in turn, speed up the weight loss process discussed later on in this book.

Reduced Time to Eat – Since you have only 8 hours to eat food every day, chances are that you will eat far less food throughout the day. And if you eat less food, you will take in fewer calories.

Fewer total calories result in a much greater chance of accomplishing a consistent calorific deficit which powerfully drives fat loss.

Eating Food Activates Inflammatory Cells In The Human Body

The #1 reason why intermittent fasting 16/8 – or fasting in general – is good for the human body is as a result of an immune cell known as monocyte, a type of granular leukocyte that functions in the ingestion of bacteria. Monocytes are secreted in order to combat infections and wounds.

Monocytes are known to be very inflammatory, and when you are injured, white blood cells cluster in order to heal the wound. But then, anytime you eat food, monocytes also congregate and stand guard in case you consume threatening microorganisms. This is particularly true when you eat or drink sugar. Monocytes also take part in the accumulation of fat tissue, thereby contributing to chronic disease.

A new study shows some of the early evidence that intermittent fasting 16/8 contributes to the calming of these inflammatory cells, thereby making them far less active. Blood samples were taken from 12 very healthy adults who undertook an intermittent fasting program for about 19 hours every day. A similar experiment was also performed on mice, and the results obtained were identical.

The team of researchers discovered that the participants' monocyte levels were amazingly low while undergoing the fast. This was an unexpected result since it was generally believed that when someone undertook intermittent fasting 16/8 if the person has an infection, the monocyte will not be able to respond to it.

According to the hunch of the lead researcher, getting well-fed daily creates a perfect storm of highly inflammatory monocytes that run on overdrive in the human body. This is the commotion that sets some individuals up for chronic diseases like heart disease, diabetes, liver issues, and so on. You should expect this sooner if you always run on sugar as your daily source of energy.

Chapter Four

How to Be Always Motivated When Undertaking Intermittent Fasting 16/8

Do you know that fasting enhances the human body's normal detoxification process by getting rid of toxins via the kidneys, colon, liver, and skin? During intermittent fasting 16/8, the body turns to stored fat and uses them for energy since no food is consumed within a stipulated period. Fasting also triggers a natural healing process inside the human body. This occurs when energy is diverted from the gastrointestinal or digestive system to metabolism and the immune system.

The benefits associated with intermittent fasting 16/8 or fasting, in general, are practically endless. However, fasting is not an easy process in any way.

Intermittent fasting 16/8, just like the detoxification of the human body, can evoke several emotions. It is often very difficult for the human body to go through withdrawals, which is why the person undertaking the fast is forced to focus on the actual hunger and the mental or physical pain that accompanies some detoxification programs. The mind often tricks you into thinking that this new eating approach is much more complicated than it really is.

Make no mistake about it: it can be incredibly hard to stay motivated during intermittent fasting 16/8. However, you need to start focusing on the remarkable transformation taking place in your body for the entire process to become easier. Your body will soon become accustomed to going without food for several hours.

Before you embark on intermittent fasting 16/8, make sure you are medically sound. Check with your physician or healthcare professional, especially if you have health issues. Any interested individual may perform intermittent fasting 16/8; however, fasting must be done under strict supervision for some of these individuals.

Focus is another aspect that plays a crucial role in the success of your intermittent fasting 16/8. This can be spiritual or some simple intentions for what you want the fast to achieve at the end of the stipulated period. This is part of what will motivate you during the fast anytime it crosses your mind to give up before reaching your set goals.

There are several ways to stay motivated while fasting; however, one of the most crucial leading up to the intermittent fast is remembering to prepare or gear up physically and spiritually for the program.

Assign a specific time frame for the intermittent fast 16/8, and then set a specific goal and be ready to stick to that goal. Make the decision that you are going to start and finish the intermittent fast 16/8. Assure yourself you are strong enough to push through and endure every pain that comes with the self-imposed program.

Set a Short-Term Goal with a Tempting Reward

Choose a tiny, achievable, and measurable goal that you can readily attain within a short period. And after you have reached that goal, reward yourself with something that has nothing to do with food in general or junk food in particular. You may reward yourself with a massage, purchase new workout clothes, go to the movies, etc.

If you make the mistake of using food as your ultimate reward, your mind will be programmed to make you always feel like you are doing yourself a disservice by depriving yourself of those foods you have categorized as rewards.

This is why it is highly essential that you choose a meaningful reward that does not involve sabotaging how far you have come along the path to a wellness lifestyle via intermittent 16/8 fasting.

Get a Fasting-Accountability Friend

According to research, enlisting an accountability friend or buddy to join you in your journey to a sound and healthy lifestyle will set you up for outstanding and remarkable success. You will end up losing a lot of weight, and you will even stick far longer with the program than you envisaged.

The accountability-buddy you choose does not have to be someone living close to you. Thanks to social media's power, you can get a Facebook friend who lives on the other side of the country or in Canada to join you in your new lifestyle journey. You may also join an online forum or community or WhatsApp group to achieve the same purpose.

Watch Videos or Read Blog Posts/Articles

All you may need to stay motivated on your journey to sound health and weight loss via intermittent fasting 16/8 is reading or watching something that inspires you.

Visit YouTube and search for videos of someone else's highly successful and completed journey towards securing the perfect body and the numerous transformations that come with it.

Google blogs that talk about intermittent fasting 16/8 as well as the benefits associated with this new approach to consuming food. Read up the journeys of successful bloggers who practiced what they preach by engaging in intermittent fasting 16/8 and the fantastic transformations within and outside their bodies.

All these will motivate you to forge ahead, and you will only have one thought in mind: if they could do it, you can, too!

Close Your Eyes, and Imagine What Your Life Will Look in the Future

Be honest with yourself; how did you feel and look before you embarked on the journey of intermittent fasting 16/8? What about the positive changes you have started experiencing? Once you have observed all these, start creating scenarios and questions around each of them.

This is a motivational tactic that practically forces you to take stock of your life just before you decided to get healthy and how worse you would have felt if you had continued down that dangerous, unhealthy path. That should be even more than enough to push you along the new and healthy path you are on.

Recognize What You Need: Sometimes a Stick, At Other Times a Carrot

Rewarding yourself when you reach a particular goal is often not as motivating as punishing yourself for not reaching that goal.

To lead a very healthy lifestyle, you have to eat well, exercise appropriately, and embark on fasts, preferably intermittent fasting

16/8. No matter how long you've believed that fasting is a punishment, the best time to completely reverse that type of thinking is now.

Always Focus on Positive Issues or Things

Alive, balanced, confident, and energetic; these are the feelings you must experience when you undertake intermittent fasting 16/8. Since you are looking for motivation, focus on a particular time before starting the journey towards sound health. Recall how good you felt about the new lifestyle.

Did you receive a glowing compliment about your skin or wake up fully rested after completing our intermittent fast. How great did you feel after completing the fast? Focus on all these positive feelings evoked by your fast.

Envision Your Healthy Future

Have you tried to picture and imagine how healthy your future will look like after undertaking the intermittent fasting 16/8? If you adhere to this lifestyle, you can visualize and recreate the feelings, images, and the sounds of specific events.

However, you should do away with any adverse outcome and focus only on positive ones. Visualize only positive thoughts of success at all times.

Take Note of the Positive Changes You Have Already Experienced

Sometimes, it may be possible not to see the progress that you have made thus far. If this is so, consider spending some time to take stock of every positive change you have experienced since you committed to an intermittent fasting 16/8 instead of looking at your lack of progress.

Take a look at your clothes and appreciate how much better the clothes fit. Do you sleep much better now? Great!

Always Be Compassionate or Tender-Hearted with Your Lovely Self

Life is fickle, and sometimes, things may just not go the way you planned for the day or week. When you are not having a successful day or week, you may employ negative self-talk and get down on yourself because you didn't meet your expectations.

However, following this route will not help you in the long run. This is not the time to be discouraged about your lack of progress. Anytime you encounter rough times in life, especially during this period of intermittent fasting 16/8, you should only be compassionate with yourself.

Form the Habit of Motivating Yourself

Many people don't know this, but motivation is a habit that can be formed. And like all habits, you need to practice it every day if you want it to become a pattern or second nature. Practice it every day and at all times.

Earmark about 15 to 20 minutes every day to think about your pre-set goals, progress, where you are presently, and where you envision yourself. Then, strive to find and make positive, meaningful affirmations. Recite them within the stipulated period in your mind, in front of your mirror, or even in the car, or better still, when you commute to work.

Chapter Five

The Science Behind Intermittent Fasting

Although there is credible scientific evidence that backs the efficacy of intermittent fasting, it is not a guaranteed or a quick fix. A leading researcher and professor of circadian biology at an institute in California has suggested – after years of studying the complex biochemical process of the human body – and supported the fact that intermittent fasting benefits human health in several ways.

As mentioned earlier in this book, there is no one way to undergo intermittent fasting. You will always come across a menu of options, and each one has its own proponent.

All intermittent fasting methods are fundamentally based on the same idea: reducing your intake of calories will result in the usage of the stored fat in your body. But what makes intermittent fasting unique is that it is far easier for people to restrict food intake or calories for a specific number of hours than for days or weeks.

Intermittent fasting 16/8 or its variant was the method utilized by the lead researcher in 2012, and it involved mice. Two genetically identical sets of rodents or mice were fed with the same diet. The diet was a lab-mice version of the typical American diet which is low in protein but high in simple sugar and fat.

Although both groups of mice were given the same diet and amount of food, one set had 24-hour access to the food while the other set of mice had access to food for only 8 hours. Mice are known to be nocturnal: they sleep during the day and only eat at night.

But the mice with 24-hour access to food started eating food during the day when they were supposed to be asleep. The other set continued to live their natural lives.

After about 18 weeks, the mice with 24-hour access to food had liver damage and showed signs of insulin resistance. But the other set did not have these conditions and they also weighed at least 28 percent less than the ones with 24-hour access to food. Bear in mind that both sets of mice consumed the same number of calories per day. The same result was obtained when the research team repeated the experiment with three different groups of mice.

Scientists have discovered that several processes that take place in the human body are linked to circadian rhythms. For instance, many people know that getting sunlight early in the mornings is beneficial to their sleep and mood. And being exposed to the blue light from laptops or cell phones at 9 pm can disrupt their night's sleep.

In the same vein, food consumed at the right time nurtures the human body while even healthy foods that are eaten at the wrong time can be referred to as junk food. It will not be used as fuel but stored as fat. Intermittent fasting or time-restricted eating gives the human body more time to use up body fat.

If you extend the fasting window and shorten your eating window, you will spend longer in this fat-burning mode of the body's metabolism. But as soon as you take in solid food again, even if it is nothing but tea or black coffee with milk and sugar, your body will switch back immediately into the other mode and start burning up the carbohydrates in the beverage and storing fat and glycogen.

So, let's say you finish eating your evening snack at around 10 pm; your body's store of glycogen will be depleted by 6 am. Your body will switch to burning fat at around that period. If you usually have breakfast at 6 am but change it to 10 am, you have successfully given your body four additional hours to utilize fat as fuel.

The same experiment performed on mice was also carried out on humans. And the same effects were discovered; the participants shed off a small amount of fat. They also experienced better sleep, less hunger at night, and were more energized in the mornings. It shows that time-restricted eating or intermittent fasting has system impact on the human body.

The best way to reap the benefits of intermittent fasting or time-restricted eating is by consuming only water during your fasting window. This means you will have to do away with coffee, herbal tea or even plain tea since all of these could affect blood chemistry. This is why they are not permitted during fasts for medical or clinical blood tests.

It is also recommended that you take plain hot water as soon as you wake up as this provides the same soothing feeling that tea does. To alert, though, you may take black coffee without adding sugar, honey, creamer or other sweeteners. One teaspoon of sugar is more than enough to double your blood sugar, so stay away from it.

You can eat breakfast after you have been awake for a couple of hours. This is because 45 minutes after you wake up, cortisol – i.e.

the stress hormone – spikes. High cortisol levels can significantly impede glucose regulation in your body. And melatonin, the hormone that prepares the human body for sleep, wears off after approximately 2 hours of staying awake.

During those first two hours, the pancreas is also waking up. This is the organ that produces the insulin your body needs to use up carbohydrates in food. This is why you should try and finish up your last meal at least 2 to 3 hours before your bedtime because that is when the melatonin starts preparing your body including the pancreas – for sleep.

Intermittent fasting isn't a silver bullet for weight loss even though it has practical advantages over several other dieting options. It is accessible and easy as most people don't know or have time to count calories. There is no need to buy certain foods, track your caloric intake or plan your meals. As long as you can estimate time and limit eating and drinking to specified eating windows, you are good to go.

For a considerably long while, many people who want to lose weight have had to change their foods or change their daily menus. Intermittent fasting or time-restricted eating has the potential to expand the factors that you can control. You may retain your menu, so all there is left is to add the timing of food to your menu.

Types of Intermittent Fasting

Intermittent fasting has subtypes, and they are as follows:

i. Time-restricted Feeding

This is virtually the same as prolonged nighttime fasting. It defines the specific hours during which you can consume food as well as hours of fasting.

ii. Prolonged Nighttime Fasting

This is the particular regimen that is extensively studied with regard to cancer, and generally involves the extension of the period between dinner and breakfast. This was likely the regular diet eaten by the primitives in the past when eating was much more challenging than and not as convenient as it is today.

The standard regimen is the 16/8 method in which food is consumed between noon and 8 pm. That is 16 hours of abstaining from and 8 hours of limitless restrictions on eating.

iii.   Short-term Fasting

There are several varieties of short-term fasting known today. For instance, with alternate-day fasting, people can alternate between days that approximately 25 percent of average calories are consumed and days with no restrictions.

Whole day fasting involves eating normally 5 days per week without any restrictions.

What Intermittent Fasting is Not

Some people are always willing to try new things or experiment with something when they learn about their numerous benefits. However, some of them balk when they hear about the myths of fasting (discussed in this book) or some principles that they are not used to.

If you belong to this group of individuals, here is what intermittent fasting 16/8 is NOT:

- Intermittent fasting 16/8 does not restrict water intake. Water does not have calories. The same can be said of calorie-free water drinks, soda, coffee, and tea.
- Intermittent fasting 16/8 does not define the type of food you should eat or not eat.
- It has nothing to do with the restriction of supplements or intake of medications.
- Intermittent fasting 16/8 does not restrict or define the number of calories you should eat when you are not fasting.

Chapter Six

6 Ways Of Undertaking Intermittent Fasting

Every method of Intermittent fasting that will be highlighted in this section can be very effective. However, it depends on the individual and how consistent they are with any of their chosen intermittent fasting protocols.

Here they are in no particular order:

1. Intermittent Fasting 16/8 Method

This is the intermittent fasting method that will be discussed majorly in this book. It involves fasting every day for at least 14 hours or at most 16 hours, thereby restriction your daily food intake window to about 8 to 10 hours.

However, during this eating window, you can fit in two or three or even more meals if you choose to. This method of fasting is also called the 'Leagains Protocol' and was made highly popular by Martin Berkhan, a fitness expert.

Undertaking this method of intermittent fasting is very easy and as simple as not eating any food or consuming calories in the form of coffee or soda after dinner, and then skipping breakfast the next day.

For instance, let's say you finish your last meal by 7 pm, and you don't touch or eat any food until noon the next day, you have technically fasted for about 16 or 17 hours.

If you are one of the individuals that get very hungry in the morning and love to eat breakfast, this intermittent fasting 16/8 method can be excruciatingly difficult for you. And this means it will take some time before your body gets used to it if you don't give up along the way. But the funny thing is that most people who skip breakfast generally undertake intermittent fasting even without knowing it.

During this period of intermittent fasting 16/8, you can drink water, coffee, tea, and other beverages with zero calories. All these help to reduce the feelings of hunger while ensuring you stay hydrated at all times.

And when the eating window arrives, make sure you eat healthy foods. This method will not work for you if you pile on an excessive number of calories by consuming loads of junk food.

2. Eat Stop Eat

This method of intermittent fasting involves fasting for 24 hours once or twice every week. It was made popular by Brad Pilon, a fitness expert, and has grown in popularity over the years.

'Eat Stop Eat' has to do with fasting from dinner on the first day and eating nothing until dinner the following day. This will result in a full 24-hour fast. You can fast from lunch to lunch or breakfast to breakfast. The result of this method of intermittent fasting remains the same.

You can still take coffee, water as well as other zero-calorie beverages during the 'Eat Stop Eat' fasting. However, eating solid foods is not permitted.

If you are undertaking the 'Eat Stop Eat' intermittent fasting method in order to lose weight, it is essential that you continue to eat normally as if you were not changing your approach to eating. In other words, eat the same amount of food you eat if you were not fasting.

The potential drawback with the 'Eat Stop Eat' intermittent fasting method is that a full 24-hour fast period can be somewhat difficult for many individuals. The best way to go about is not to go all-in but start with, say 15-16 hours, and then work upward from there.

3. The 5:2 Diet

The 5:2 diet is a method of intermittent fasting that involves eating normally for 5 days of the week while restricting the intake of calories to about 500-600 for the remaining 2 days of the week. On fasting days, it is highly recommended that men eat 600 calories while women can eat up to 500 calories.

This method is also known as the 'Fast Diet' and was made popular by Michael Mosley, a British journalist.

For instance, you can eat every day of the week except Sundays and Wednesdays. For these 2 days, you eat tiny meals of about 300 calories each for men and 250 calories each for women.

Critics will be quick to point out that there are virtually no studies that test the efficacy of the 5:2 diet itself, despite the existence of numerous benefits of intermittent fasting.

4. The Warrior Diet

The Warrior Diet is the brainchild of a fitness expert known as Ori Hofmkler. This method of intermittent fasting involves eating relatively small amounts of vegetables and raw fruits during the day and eating only one very huge meal at night.

In basic terms, you fast all through the day and then have a feast at night within a 4-hour eating window.

This particular diet's food choices are very similar to that of the paleo diet, and it is one of those to include this form of intermittent fasting.

5. Alternative-day fasting

This method of intermittent fasting involves fasting every other day. But then, there are more than a few versions of this particular product. Some of them allow participants to consume up to 500 calories during fasting days.

Several test-tube studies have shown the numerous health benefits of intermittent fasting using some versions of this method of fasting.

A full fast every other day seems somewhat extreme to some individuals as well as health professionals. This is why it is generally not recommended for beginners or those who have never fasted intermittently.

If you must follow this method of intermittent fasting, you should be ready to go to bed very hungry several times every week. This is not going to be pleasant for you in any way and is usually unsustainable – for most people – in the long term.

6. Spontaneous Meal Skipping

You do not need to follow any structured intermittent fasting approach or plan in order to reap some of its remarkable health benefits. You can skip meals once in a while, especially when you don't feel hungry or discover you are way too busy to cook and eat.

Many individuals erroneously subscribe to the myth that people have to eat every few hours or else they will slip into 'starvation mode' or end up losing lots of muscles. This is not the case.

The human body is super-equipped to deal with extended periods of famine, so missing a meal or two occasionally will not do any harm to it. So, if you discover that you are not too hungry one day, consider skipping breakfast. You may eat a healthy lunch or a heavy dinner.

You can also do a short fast if you need to travel and cannot find anything good to eat at the venue. Skipping a meal or two when you feel like it is known as a spontaneous intermittent fast.

On a final note for this section, if you want to try any of the intermittent fasting methods outline here, bear in mind that the quality of the diet you consume is vital. You are not expected to binge on junk foods during the eating window, or your goal for following this new approach to eating may not be met.

Finally, make sure you are certified fit and capable of undertaking intermittent fast by a healthcare professional before embarking on the program.

Benefits of Intermittent Fasting 16/8

Researchers and enthusiasts have studied the benefits of intermittent fasting 16/8 for decades. Many of these findings and studies end with inconclusive or contradictory outcomes.

Nevertheless, intermittent fasting 16/8 – and other forms of intermittent fasting – provide the following health benefits that should never be missed.

-Blood Sugar Regulation

According to a new, extensive study conducted by a team of researchers working at University of Adelaide, it has been discovered intermittent fasting 16/8 – otherwise known as time-restricted eating – may help in regulating blood glucose sugar levels among individuals who are highly at risk of type 2 diabetes.

Fasting was shown to significantly improve blood sugar or glycemic responses in men who are at a very high risk of developing the polygenic disease, regardless of how much food or the type of food they consumed.

Most people that follow this approach to eating know that more extended fasting periods significantly increase the human body's ability to deal with or manage larger volumes of food.

Intermittent Fasting 16/8 Put to the Test

The journal, 'Obesity' reported that the team of researchers analyzed 15 at-risk individuals for 2 seven-day test periods. The men did not deviate from their usual diet; however, they limited their daily intake of food to a 9-hour period. This means they ate between 8 am and 5 pm for 1 week or between noon and 9 pm for a week.

Every participant carried a continuous glucose monitor were readily assessed for glucose tolerance after a standard meal both at the start as well as the end of the experiment.

The team of researchers reported that intermittent eating 16/8 significantly improved glucose control, regardless of when the participants choose to stop eating.

Significant Improvements Acknowledged

One of the participants followed his usual diet between 9:30 am and 7:30 pm over 8 weeks. According to this person, the intermittent fasting 16/8 was somewhat challenging but became manageable when the body started adapting to the new style of eating. Fasting blood tolerance improved noticeably and even changed from 'high risk' to 'normal.' This occurred without having to change any of the foods they like to eat.

These findings are expected to be replicated in future studies that involve more participants and carried out over an extended period before drawing full conclusions.

This early result has, however, shown some promise when it comes to controlling blood glucose. A much larger study will be required in order to determine the effectiveness of this eating pattern.

-Highly Beneficial for Type 2 Diabetic Patients

Type 2 diabetes is a polygenic or metabolic disease that is generally characterized by resistance to insulin. Insulin is that hormone that is secreted by beta cells present in the pancreas.

When you consume food, especially carbohydrate-laden foods, your blood sugar level will rise considerably as the food undergoes digestions.

Insulin will obtain sugar from your blood – i.e. blood glucose – and transport it to several areas of your body that need it, including your brain. Insulin resistance is a health condition that occurs when the body responds in a dysfunctional to insulin. This response makes the human body far less effective at transporting sugar or glucose from the blood to the human brain. This ends up resulting in chronically high blood sugar.

Another study revealed that intermittent fasting 16/8 decreases fasting blood sugar by 3-6 percent and also decreases insulin by 20-31 percent. This is why intermittent fasting 16/8 is considered the best option for people with type 2 diabetes to adopt from time to time because it is easy to follow and also sustainable.

-Fat Loss And Weight Loss

Intermittent fasting 16/8 entails eating within stipulated hours or eating windows. This generally implies that people who undertake this style of intermittent fasting will significantly minimize the number of calories they take in or consume. This will also have the additional benefit of boosting metabolism.

According to a study conducted in 2017, intermittent fasting 16/8 results in a more significant or greater fat loss and weight loss in people with obesity than those who follow calorie-restrictive diets.

Another research conducted as far back as 2016 has reported that individuals who engaged in intermittent fasting 16/8 strictly for 8 weeks while engaging passionately in resistance training showed a marked decrease in fat mass. These participants were able to maintain their muscle mass throughout.

But in contrast to the study mentioned above, another study carried out in 2017 hardly found any notable difference in weight loss between participants that passionately practiced intermittent fasting. This was conducted in the form of alternate-day fasting instead of the intermittent fasting 16/8 method as against those who minimized their overall intake of calories. The dropout was also predominantly high among the participants that engaged in intermittent fasting 16/8.

-Longevity And Body Cleansing

Animal studies indicate that intermittent fasting 16/8 may help animals to live longer than they should. For instance, one study showed that temporary but repeated intermittent fasting significantly increase d the lifespan of female rodents or mice.

According to the National Institute on Aging have stated that scientists are still unable to explain precisely how intermittent fasting lengthens life span, even after decades of dedicated research. And this is why they cannot readily confirm the long-term benefits of this unique approach to eating.

Human studies in this particular area are severely limited, and so the potential benefits of intermittent fasting 16/8 for human longevity remains unknown.

-Reduced Oxidative Stress

The human body naturally produces what is known as 'free radicals,' which are natural byproducts of human metabolism. However, excess free radicals can be toxic to the human body. This can bring about untold damage to tissue and cells via a process known as oxidative stress.

Studies have revealed that intermittent fasting 16/8 may be able to improve the human body's resistance to oxidative stress.

Oxidative stress is known to speed up aging and is also linked with the onslaught of a variety of chronic diseases. Antioxidants which can be obtained from the consumption of vegetables and fruits can counteract oxidative damage. They are also powerful enough to prevent free radical damage to your cells, DNA, and proteins.

-Increased autophagy

Intermittent fasting 16/8 has been scientifically shown to bring on autophagy which is a process that causes cells to recycle themselves by getting rid of unnecessary waste.

-Prevention Of Life-Threatening Diseases

According to advocates of intermittent fasting 16/8, it is believed that this method of fasting helps to prevent debilitating diseases and health conditions such as type 2 diabetes, cancers, neurodegenerative diseases, and heart conditions.

Research about these claims is severely limited. Nevertheless, according to a 2014 review, intermittent fasting 16/8 shows remarkable promise as an excellent alternative to conventional calorie restriction for weight loss and type 2 diabetes risk reduction in people who are obese or overweight. Additional research in this area is also crucial in order to reach or draw reliable conclusions.

A study in 2018 indicates that intermittent fasting 16/8 helps to reduce blood pressure in obese adults, in addition to weight loss. Intermittent fasting also brings down fasting glucose by up 6 percent in people with prediabetes, though this particular impact is not felt or discovered in healthy individuals. It has also been shown to significantly minimize fasting insulin by at least 11 percent and up to 57 percent after approximately 3 to 24 weeks of intermittent fasting.

Intermittent fasting 16/8 has been shown to protect memory and learning. It also slows down diseases that may affect the brain. There will be a bit more discussion about this remarkable benefit to the human brain later on in this book.

An annual review in 2017 notes that intermittent fasting 16/8 reduces the risk of cancer and nonalcoholic fatty liver disease, based on animal research.

-Improved Cardiovascular Health

One of the leading causes of death globally is heart disease. Numerous health makers such as blood pressure, inflammatory markers, LDL cholesterol levels, triglyceride levels, and blood sugar levels are major risk factors that healthcare professionals use in order to accurately predict and diagnose an individual's risk of heart diseases. For instance, a high amount of fat in the blood or high triglyceride levels is strongly linked with an increased risk of cardiac or heart disease. Intermittent fasting 16/8 has been shown to improve several of these risk factors in numerous studies greatly.

Nevertheless, more research is highly required in order to determine whether caloric restriction or intermittent fasting 16/8, which really improves these risk factors. Intermittent fasting 16/8 helps to promote weight loss, and this helps to bring down triglyceride levels. This is why it is somewhat difficult for researchers to distinguish whether it is weight loss per se or intermittent fasting 16/8 which is a consequence of meal timing, which in turn, improves heart diseases risk factors.

-Boosts Cognition And Focus

Emerging studies have revealed that intermittent fasting 16/8 may contribute to the improvement of brain health.

A study carried out on group of mice showed that intermittent fasting 16/8 was able to substantially increase the development and growth of new nerve cells which are highly beneficial for brain health.

Another research has also revealed that intermittent fasting 16/8 increases BDNF (brain-derived neurotrophic factor). This is a protein that upregulates the production of brain cells via a process that is known as neurogenesis. Brain-derived neurotrophic factor enhances the maturation and integrity of nerve cells.

Lower BNDF levels have been said to play a crucial role in the pathophysiology of depression. This is an indication that boosting BDNF via intermittent fasting 16/8 could improve symptoms of depression.

However, depression is a complex field, and clinical trials that link intermittent fasting 16/8 and depression are hard to come by.

-Increased Growth Hormone

According to research, short-term intermittent fasting 16/8 can significantly increase growth hormone levels five-fold. Higher levels of growth hormone are generally required during fasting periods for several reasons, such as the preservation of muscle mass and increased energy availability.

Higher growth hormone levels are significantly associated with increased muscle mass, decreased aging, increased strength, as well as lower body fat percentage.

Chapter Seven

Drawbacks of Intermittent Fasting 16/8

Intermittent fasting 16/8 has been linked with side effects and risks. This is why it is not for everyone, and anyone who wishes to undertake this style of fasting should consult their physicians.

The potential drawbacks of intermittent fasting 16/8 includes:

- Heartburn or reflux due to overeating
- Eating unhealthy foods or overeating during the eating window as a result of excessive hunger.
- Weakness, hunger, and general tiredness or fatigue during the beginning stages of the new lifestyle.

Intermittent fasting 16/8 is also considered more beneficial to men than women. This is because research carried out on animals appears to suggest that intermittent fasting 16/8 could negatively and significantly affect fertility. But there is a right way to engage in intermittent fasting 16/8 that will not affect the hormonal balances of women.

Nothing is taught about healthy eating, and this could end up, resulting in excessive calorie intake. This is highly detrimental to your overall health and can cause the very thing you are battling against, which is weight gain.

Many beginners make the mistake of taking intermittent fasting 16/8 to the extreme. All meals are expected to cover a wide range of nutrient-rich foods in order to ensure a balanced diet.

Moreover, since you are expected to eat within a specified time frame, intermittent fasting 16/8 still instills that dieting mindset that is common nowadays. If you believe you are following a so-called diet, you are far less likely to want to follow through to the very end.

This particular eating pattern has absolutely nothing to do with the theory of calories in equals calories out. If you eat more calories than you burn off, i.e. without engaging in intense physical activities, etc. and irrespective of when you eat them, you will ultimately put on a lot of weight. And you will be disappointed and probably claim that intermittent fasting 16/8 does not work for you, whereas the reverse is the case.

If you have a very long history of eating disorders like anorexia, it is best to avoid intermittent fasting 16/8. According to the National Eating Disorders Association, intermittent fasting 16/8 is a risk factor for eating disorders.

Restricting your intake of food to just 8 hours per day can cause those who engage in the practice to eat even more than usual during the eating window in a vain attempt to make up for the hours spent fasting. This may ultimately result in digestive problems, weight gain, as well as the development and promotion of unhealthy eating habits.

Intermittent fasting 16/8 may also not be too suitable for you if you have a history of anxiety and depression. Studies have shown that short-term or temporary calorie-restriction may relieve depression. But chronic restriction of calories can have the opposite – and highly unpleasant – effect on the human body. Additional research, however, is required to fully understand these findings and their implications.

Pregnant Women And Breastfeeding Mothers

Intermittent fasting 16/8 is also highly unsuitable to pregnant or breastfeeding women. This is because during any of these periods, you will be eating for two, and engaging in intermittent fasting 16/8 will deprive you and your baby of essential nutrients, food as well as much-needed energy when you need it. Those who are also trying to conceive are not encouraged to try intermittent fasting 16/8. The National Institute on Aging has also concluded that evidence to recommend any form of diet to older adults is grossly insufficient.

Once again, those trying the intermittent fasting 16/8 method or any other type of fast for that matter, should first of all talk to their healthcare professionals or physician, especially if they are on medications. You should stay away from intermittent fasting 16/8 if you have:

- A history of eating disorders like anorexia
- An underlying health condition, such as low blood pressure, diabetes, etc.
- A history of mental health complications

If you aren't up to 18 years of age or are underweight, you should stay away from intermittent fasting 16/8. If you experience any adverse or harmful effects as a result of engaging in intermittent fasting 16/8, you should see a medical doctor immediately.

Stress-sensitive people

Intermittent fasting 16/8 puts a lot of stress on the human body. Increased stress is associated with the absence of food. And one of the primary reasons why intermittent fasting 16/8 is highly beneficial is due to its stressfulness, which is similar to the benefits enjoyed via workouts.

The stress brought on by workouts is exceptionally stressful for the human body. However, the body soon recovers and becomes much more resilient to that stress. Intermittent fasting 16/8 works similarly; it is an adaptive response known as 'hormesis.'

But then, too much stress, especially for people who are very sensitive to stress, can be very harmful. Intermittent fasting 16/8 crucially increases stress hormones such as adrenaline and cortisol. Increased amounts of stress hormones in the human body results can significantly boost energy levels. And over time, chronic stress can be painfully detrimentally.

No doubt, you will be stressed for other reasons as a result of day-to-day living, and adding the stress associated with intermittent fasting 16/8 can make things decidedly worse for you.

You should try intermittent fasting 16/8; however, consider starting very slow if you find that you are very sensitive to stress.

Diabetes

Evidence about the efficacy of intermittent fasting 16/8 in diabetes prevention abound. However, this time-restricting approach to eating may be very unsuitable for individuals with this debilitating health condition.

Intermittent fasting 16/8 is not for people with type 1 diabetes. Some people with type 2 diabetes or prediabetes may embark on the program. But this may be done under the supervision of a medical doctor or healthcare professional.

This is why it is generally advised that people with type 2 diabetes who want to try the intermittent fasting 16/8 method should see their physician before they make any changes to their established or prescribed eating habits. Another reason for seeing a medical doctor before undertaking the program is that doses of medications will need to be adapted for people with diabetes.

Chapter Eight

Benefits of Intermittent Fasting to the Human Brain

Intermittent fasting 16/8 has been proven to reduce inflammation, losing weight, and – in this section – supercharges the human brain. Although more research is required in some aspects in order to garner additional proofs of the effect of intermittent fasting 16/8 on the human body, recent studies have revealed that this method of food restriction has profound benefits for the brain.

In this section, you will discover the exciting and surprising benefits of intermittent fasting 16/8 to the human brain. Here they are in no particular order:

Intermittent Fasting Reduces Inflammation

Intermittent fasting 16/8 has shown via in-depth studies to reduce inflammation, or inflammatory reaction which end up reducing damage to brain cells as waste in the brain are eliminated. Excessive inflammation is the root cause of several chronic diseases that many individuals face today, including dementia, Alzheimer's, diabetes, obesity, and so much more.

Intermittent fasting has been proven to reduce inflammation in the following ways:

- **Insulin Sensitivity**: Fasting has been clinically proven to deal with insulin resistance. When the human body becomes very resistant to insulin, glucose, and insulin start to build up in the blood, which results in inflammation. Intermittent fasting allows the human body to take a good break.

  And since there is no food to digest at expected meal times, the human body uses up all its sugar stores. Insulin levels in the blood will begin to drop, thereby allowing the body to become re-sensitized to insulin again.

- **Autophagy**: Autophagy is a biological process the human body undergoes in which damaged and old cells in the body are destroyed, and new ones are created. You can think of it as the body cleaning off rust and then cleansing itself. It is this process the human body undergoes in order to repair itself and facilitates communication in the brain.

  If damaged or old cells remain in the human body, they can bring about inflammation. Intermittent fasting efficiently stimulates autophagy, thereby helping the human body to cleanse itself, which culminates in reduced inflammation.

- **Ketones**: During fasting, the human body uses up all its sugar stores. And when there are no more sugars to burn, the body turns to fat for fuel. And when fats are broken down, it creates what is known as 'ketones.' One of the most popular and abundant ketones 'β-hydroxybutyrate' works by blocking part of the immune system that is fully responsible for the regulation of inflammatory disorders like Alzheimer's disease, arthritis, etc.

It Creates Even More Brain Cells

Do you know you can create more brain cells – thereby significantly boosting your brainpower – by undertaking intermittent fasting? According to a professor of Neurology at Johns Hopkins University, fasting has been shown to boost rates of neurogenesis in the human brain. Neurogenesis is a process that involves the growth as well as the development of nerve tissues and new brain cells.

According to confirmed clinical studies, higher rates of neurogenesis are linked to increased brain action, mood, memory, and focus. One distinct study even revealed that intermittent fasting 16/8 considerably stimulated the development and production of new brain cells.

Intermittent Fasting Increases BDNF

Fasting, in general, has been shown to substantially boost the production of a vital protein known as BDNF, the so-called 'Miracle Grow' for the human brain. Deficits in this essential protein have been associated with cognitive problems during aging, such as dementia.

Studies have revealed that BDNF plays a crucial role in neuroplasticity which allows the human brain to adapt and continue to change from time to time. It makes the brain much more resilient to undue stress and quite adaptable to change.

BDNF has also been proven to help in the production of new brain cells, the stimulation of synapses and new connections as well as the protection of your brain cells. All these culminate in the boosting of your memory, improving your mood, and learning.

It Supercharges Your Energy

Intermittent fasting boosts mitochondrial biogenesis, which is the creation of new mitochondria. Mitochondria serve as the batteries of your cells. And each cell is filled with hundreds of mitochondria designed to power the cells to do their respective jobs. Their primary assignment is to take any food you eat and convert it to energy.

The presence of mitochondria in the brain gives you more brainpower, providing longer-lasting energy.

Intermittent Fasting Boosts HGH (Human Growth Hormone)

The first thing that quickly comes to mind when someone hears 'Human Growth Hormone' or HGH is the image of a bodybuilder using the hormone to build great muscles. This may not be far from the truth, but in reality, the human growth hormone sourced from the outside is usually not recommended for a wide variety of health reasons.

Although the human growth hormone from an exogenous – i.e. outside – source is not the best for your body, it has been discovered that it possesses incredibly powerful, longevity and anti-aging benefits. HGH has also been proven to provide neuroprotection, improve cognition, and increase neurogenesis.

One particular study even showed that the human growth hormone displayed a neuroprotective effect, preserving your brain performance as well as your brain health.

Intermittent fasting 16/8 naturally boost HGH levels in the body, which end up providing repair, healthy, longevity, and neuroprotective benefits.

Burns Fat Instead Of Sugar

You already know what happens when you go on a fast; the body turns to fat when carbohydrates or sugars are depleted from the stores, and none is accessible or available via food.

Fat is actually a cleaner and better source of fuel than carbohydrates. It produces much more energy per gram than carbohydrates generate. Moreover, fat produces far less free radicals – which are the culprits that cause inflammation in the body – than carbohydrates do.

When your cell batteries or mitochondria use up ketones (fat) or even carbohydrates to produce energy, the waste that is created in the process are free radicals.

Free radicals bring about oxidative stress to the human body and are believed to be behind several chronic and neurodegenerative diseases that are faced by humanity today.

The intermittent fasting 16/8 method forces your brain to use ketones – instead of carbohydrates or sugar – which is a much more efficient and cleaner fuel for the human brain.

Chapter Nine

Fasting and Cancer

Over the past few years, multiple, extensive studies have been published, which shows the link between intermittent fasting and cancer.

Cancer involves uncontrolled cell growth and negative cell changes. Autophagy – which is a process promoted by intermittent fasting – helps to get rid of cellular waste. This cellular process involves the breaking down of part of cells for reuse later on. And it is vital for the proper maintenance of cell function. It also helps in defending cells in the human body. It is now known that autophagy plays a crucial role in the prevention and treatment of cancer.

But dysregulated autophagy, on the other hand, is linked with a host of chronic diseases including cancer.

Animal studies conducted recently, as well as a handful of preliminary human trials, have that intermittent fasting engenders a decrease in cancer growth rates. The studies correctly indicate that the following effects are as a result of intermittent fasting:

- A balanced nutritional intake

- A decrease in blood glucose production
- An increase in the production of tumor-killing cells
- Triggering of stem cells in order to regenerate

In one particular study of intermittent fasting, fasting was shown to substantially reverse the progression of type 2 diabetes and obesity in mice. Obesity has been considered one of the significant risk factors for cancer.

In a study conducted in 2016, it was revealed that a combination of chemotherapy and fasting remarkably slowed the progression of skin cancer and breast cancer. These innovatively combined treatment methods caused the human body to produce generous amounts of CLPs (common lymphoid progenitor cells) as well as tumor-infiltrating lymphocytes. Common lymphoid progenitor cells herald lymphocytes, i.e. the white blood cells that move into a tumor and are notorious for killing off tumors.

The same 2016 study also noted that intermittent fasting or short-term starvation made cancer cells visibly sensitive to chemotherapy. Normal cells, on the other hand, were protected. The program also stimulated the production of stem cells. It is, therefore, now believed that intermittent fasting can remarkably boost the immune system in order to help combat cancer that is already present.

According to some researchers, intermittent fasting vastly improves the responses of people with cancer to chemotherapy because the following occurs:

- It protects blood from the harmful or adverse effects of chemotherapy.
- It stimulates cellular regeneration.
- It dramatically reduces the overall impact of fallouts or side effects such as nausea, fatigue, cramps, and headaches.

A study carried out in 2018 found that fasting markedly improved the quality of life of individuals undergoing chemotherapy for ovarian cancer or breast cancer. The study involved the use of a 60-hour fasting period, which started 36 hours before the commencement of chemotherapy treatment.

The results showed that the participants that fasted during chemotherapy reported a much higher tolerance to cancer treatment or therapy. They also experienced much fewer chemotherapy-related fallouts and enjoyed higher energy levels when compared to the participants who did not fast.

A study performed in 2014 examined fasting to understand how it produces cancer-fighting effects in mice stem cells if any. Stem cells are essential due to their remarkable regenerative abilities.

It was revealed that fasting for 2-4 days might considerably protect stem cells against the unfavorable effect of chemotherapy on the immune system. Fasting has also been proven to activate the stem cells of the immune system in order to repair or renew themselves. Fasting does not only reduce severe damage to cells, but it also revitalizes white blood cells while replacing the damaged ones.

White blood cells are designed to combat infection and kill off cells that may cause any disease. When the level of white blood cell levels in the blood drop drastically, no thanks to chemotherapy, it adversely affects the immune system. This makes it more difficult for that individual to fight infections.

The number of white blood cells generally decreases during fasting. But as the fasting cycle concludes – depending on the type of fasting you are engaged in – and the body receives food, the levels of white blood cells rise rapidly.

To round up this section, both short and prolonged fasting periods have shown promising results in the fight against cancer itself as well as cancer prevention, according to numerous studies over the years. However, it remains unclear which particular fasting schedule generates the best results.

Any individual who is overly curious about fasting and its efficacy as well as how it would be of immense benefit to them during their cancer treatment should speak with their healthcare specialist.

Chapter Ten

Intermittent Fasting and Your Diet

Eating while undertaking intermittent fasting can be extremely confusing. And this is because intermittent fasting is not a diet plan but a unique approach to eating or eating pattern. Most people that attempt intermittent fasting aim to lose excess weight by burning off body fat. But the diet they stick to, especially during their eating windows – for those undertaking intermittent fasting 16/8 – can mar their efforts.

Intermittent fasting may tell you when to eat, but it does not specify what foods you should include in your diet. This complete lack of distinct or clear-cut dietary guidelines often gives a very false impression that you can eat anything and whatever you want. This can cause lots of problems with choosing the right type of food to eat.

As mentioned earlier, a lack of dietary guidelines can also sabotage your entire weight loss effort. A third possibility – and an unpleasant one – is that you are very likely to be overnourished or undernourished.

Choosing the Best Foods for Your Intermittent Fast

Eating during intermittent fasting is much more about staying healthy than rapidly losing excess weight. This is why it is highly necessary to choose and eat nutrient-rich foods such as lean proteins, veggies, healthy fats, etc.

Here is what the intermittent fasting food list should have:

For Carbs

According to a scientific body, the Dietary Guidelines for Americans, 45-65 percent of your everyday calories should be obtained from carbs (carbohydrate).

It has been established before now that carbs are the primary source of energy for the human body. They come in numerous forms, and the most common ones are starch, sugar, and fiber. The other two sources of energy are fat and protein.

Carbs are notorious for causing weight gain. But in reality, not all carbs are culprits as some of them are not inherently fattening. The quantity and type of carbs you consume will determine whether or not you will gain a lot of weight. This is why you should go for foods that are loaded with starch and fiber but extremely low in sugar in sugar.

A study in 2015 reveals that eating up to 30 grams of fiber every day can improve glucose levels, cause weight loss, and significantly lower blood pressure.

It is never an uphill challenge to get up to 30 grams of fiber every day. You can quickly get it by eating an egg sandwich, chicken and black peas enchiladas, Mediterranean barley with chickpeas, and apple with peanut butter.

Here is the intermittent fasting food list for carbs:

- Sweet potatoes
- Apples
- Mangoes
- Avocado
- Oats
- Beetroots
- Kidney beans
- Carrots

- Quinoa
- Berries
- Brown rice
- Pears
- Chia seeds
- Broccoli
- Chickpeas
- Brussels sprouts
- Almonds

For Proteins

The Recommended Dietary Allowance (RDA) for protein is 0.8 grams of protein per kilogram of body weight. However, your requirements may vary considerably, depending on your level of activity and fitness goals.

Protein helps you to lose excess weight by minimizing energy intake, boosting metabolism, and increasing satiety. Increased protein intake, when combined with strength training, helps to build muscle. When you have more muscle in your body than fat, metabolism will naturally increase. This is because muscle burns even more calories than fat ever will.

One of the recent studies on intermittent fasting and overall health has suggested that having more muscles in the legs can assist in reducing the formation of belly fat in healthy individuals.

Here is the intermittent fasting for proteins

- Seafood
- Eggs
- Legumes and beans
- Fish and poultry
- Nuts and seeds
- Soy
- Whole grains

For A Healthy Gut

A growing body of scientific or clinical evidence indicates that your gut health is crucial to your overall health. For those who do not know, your gut is home to several billions of bacteria commonly known as the microbiota.

These are the bacteria that affect digestion, gut health, and mental health. They are also known to play critical roles in several chronic disorders. This is why you should consider taking great care of these tiny bugs in your tummy, especially if you are undertaking intermittent fasting.

Here is the intermittent fasting food list for healthy guts:

- All vegetables
- Kimchi
- Miso
- Fermented vegetables
- Kefir
- Tempeh
- Kombucha
- Sauerkraut

These foods, in addition to ensuring your gut stays healthy, also help you to lose weight during intermittent fasting. They also assist with the following:

- Increase the excretion of ingested fat via stools

- Decrease the overall absorption of fat from the gut
- Reduce food intake

For Fats

The Dietary Guidelines for Americans (2015-2020) have made it known that fats should contribute 20 percent to 35 percent of your everyday calories. Saturated fat, however, should not contribute over 10 percent of daily calories.

The truth is that fats can be very good, threatening, or somewhat in-between; it depends primarily on the type. For instance, trans fat is known to increase inflammation considerably while reducing the levels of 'good' cholesterol and increasing 'bad' cholesterol levels in the human body. They are generally found in baked goods and fried foods.

Saturated fats increase the risk of heart disease. However, expert opinions differ significantly on this. For this reason, it is often highly recommended to eat saturated fats in moderation. High amounts of this type of fat can be found in red meat, baked goods, coconut oil, and whole milk.

Healthy fats, on the hand, include both monounsaturated and polyunsaturated fats. These fats help to minimize the risk of lower blood pressure, heart disease, as well as the blood levels of fats.

Excellent sources of healthy fats include peanut oil, olive oil, soybean oils, sunflower oil, canola oil, and safflower oil.

Here's the intermittent fasting food list for fats:

- Fatty fish
- Avocados
- Nuts
- Whole eggs
- Cheese
- Chia seeds
- Full-fat yogurt
- Extra virgin olive oil (EVOO)

Hydration

The National Academies of Sciences, Engineering, and Medicine has stated that the daily fluid requirement is:

- 3.7 liters (approximately 15.5 cups) for men

- 2.7 liters (about 11.5 cups) for women

Fluids include water, foods as well as drinks that contain water. It is vital to stay hydrated during intermittent fasting, as it is very critical to your overall health. Dehydration can trigger headaches, dizziness, and extreme tiredness. It can also make any side effect of fasting worse or even severe.

Here's the intermittent fasting list for hydration:

- Water
- Watermelon
- Sparkling water
- Peaches
- Oranges
- Cantaloupe
- Black coffee or tea
- Cucumber
- Strawberries
- Plain yogurt
- Celery
- Skim milk

- Tomatoes
- Lettuce

Interestingly – and somewhat shockingly – drinking lots of water also contributes to weight loss. According to a 2016 review study, adequate hydration helps you to lose weight via:

- Increasing body fat burning
- Decreasing food intake or appetite

Exclude these Foods from Intermittent Fasting

Here are some foods you should exclude during your intermittent fast:

- Refined grains
- Processed foods
- Candy bars
- Alcoholic beverages
- Trans-fat
- Processed meat
- Sugar-sweetened beverages

Intermittent fasting continues to be studied as one of the most potent and highly effective eating patterns for weight loss. Eating healthy, therefore, is vital in order to prevent nutritional deficiencies. This is why you should take foods such as veggies, lean proteins, fruits, seeds, etc.

And there is nothing wrong with drinking water while undertaking intermittent fasting.

Chapter Eleven

Is Breakfast the Most Important Meal of the Whole Day?

You have probably heard that the healthiest and fittest people in the world don't skip breakfast. And one of the most well-worn phrases our parents used to drum in our ears is that breakfast is the most important specialty of every day. Many of us grew up believing that skipping the first meal of the day is nothing but a dietary sin.

But in reality, breakfast is the meal that is used to break our overnight fast. According to a dietician, the human body utilizes a lot of energy stores for repair and growth throughout the night. Eating a well-balanced breakfast helps to boost energy as well as the calcium and protein used overnight.

However, there is a widely circulated disagreement over whether breakfast should be knocked off its top spot in the pecking order of meals or let it be. The rising popularity of numerous fasting diets is also making many to take a second look at the sugar content of cereal as well as the involvement of the food industry in pro-breakfast research. There is even an academic claim that breakfast is acutely dangerous to one's health.

What is, therefore, the reality? Is breakfast truly the most important meal or specialty of the day or is it a marketing gimmick – that lasted for decades – by cereal companies?

Researched aspects of breakfast have been linked to obesity, though scientists have numerous and different theories about why a relationship exists between the two.

According to a study in the United States in which the health data of 50,000 individuals were analyzed over 7 years, it was discovered that those who took breakfast as the largest meal of the day were highly likely to have lower BMI (body mass index) than those who ate large lunches or dinners.

The researchers also argued that breakfast helps to reduce daily calorie intake, increases satiety, and improves the quality of people's diet. This is because most breakfast foods are high in nutrients and fiber, which enhance insulin sensitivity at subsequent meals.

A review of 10 studies in 2016 looked at the relationship between breakfast and weight management. It concluded that there is limited evidence refuting or supporting the argument that breakfast influences food intake or weight gain.

For Mental Clarity

Believe it or not, your brain is a big deal as it is in charge of keeping your lungs breathing, your heart beating, and allows you to think, feel, and move. This is why it is a great and rewarding idea to keep your brain working at peak condition.

This also implies that the food you should eat to contribute to the health of your brain and enhance mental clarity and tasks such as concentration and memory.

The following foods can be consumed at breakfast for mental clarity:

- Black coffee
- Broccoli
- Turmeric
- Blueberries
- Nuts
- Dark chocolate
- Pumpkin seeds
- Oranges
- Green tea

- Eggs

For Weight Loss

When trying to lose weight, only a handful of individuals know that breakfast can set the perfect tone for the remaining hours of the day. If you consume the wrong foods at breakfast, it will amplify your cravings, thereby setting you up for failure long before the day even rolls on.

But when you fill yourself with the right foods, cravings will be curbed, and you will feel full until lunchtime, thereby minimizing snacking and easing weight loss.

These healthy breakfast foods will help you to lose weight:

- Eggs
- Bananas
- Yogurt
- Nuts
- Oatmeal
- Wheat germ
- Grapefruits

- Flaxseeds
- Smoothies
- Black coffee
- Green tea
- Chia seeds
- Kiwis

So, is breakfast the most important meal of the day? The answer is, it depends as everyone starts their day differently. The #1 key is to be mindful of not over-emphasizing any particular meal but look at how you eat throughout the day.

Breakfast may be most important for individuals that are hungry as soon as they wake up. For instance, research has revealed that people with diabetes and pre-diabetes may discover that they have much better concentration after having a lower-GI breakfast such as porridge. Porridge is usually broken down very slowly and causes a gradual rise in blood sugar levels.

Breakfast is not the only meal that you should get right. Getting regular meals all day long is much more critical in order to maintain blood sugar levels throughout the day as this helps to control hunger and weight levels.

Make sure the breakfast you take is well-balanced at all times.

Combining Specific Diets and Intermittent Fasting

A school of thought believe that combining intermittent fasting with specific diets such as a vegetarian diet or keto diet is much more effective for weight loss than undertaking intermittent fasting only.

If you want to give a combination of intermittent fasting and the keto diet, for instance, remember to add the following in the food list:

For protein, i.e. 20 percent of your daily calories.

- Eggs
- Seeds and nuts
- Soy
- Seafood
- Whole grains
- Fish and poultry
- Legumes and beans

- Dairy products like yogurt, milk, and cheese

For fats, i.e. 75 percent of your daily calories.

- Full-fat yogurt
- Nuts
- Chia seeds
- Whole egg
- Cheese
- Dark chocolate
- Avocado
- Fatty fish
- Extra virgin olive oil

For carbs, i.e. 5 percent of your daily calories.

- Oats
- Quinoa
- Brown rice
- Sweet potatoes
- Beetroots

Vegetarians can also engage in intermittent fasting. Combine intermittent fasting with vegetarian diet viz.:

For Carbs

- Quinoa
- Oats
- Sweet potatoes
- Apples
- Bananas
- Beetroots
- Brown rice
- Broccoli
- Berries
- Brussels sprouts
- Chia seeds
- Kidney beans
- Pears
- Chickpeas

For Fats

- Avocados
- Full-fat yogurt
- Extra virgin olive oil
- Cheese
- Nuts
- Dark chocolate
- Chia seeds

For Protein

- Soy
- Seed and nuts
- Dairy products, e.g. yogurt, cheese etc.
- Whole grains

Chapter Twelve

Correct Mindset

If you can't set the right mindset, you will not be able to achieve the results that intermittent fasting provides. Many individuals have failed to achieve these results, and it has all been linked to not being able to set the right mindset. And so they end up quitting long before they even start observing the changes they crave for.

The truth is that intermittent fasting should not and cannot be seen as a one-time program or a once-in-a-lifetime thingy. You have to be very consistent and even make it part of your lifestyle. Fasting is also not meant to be a quick fix or punish you; it is intended to reward your body with enough time to repair itself and heal.

You must also be very clear and specific about your goals. For instance, why are you doing intermittent fasting? Are you doing it in order to lose weight or just to stay healthy? You may be engaging in intermittent fasting 16/8 in order to help your body avoid insulin resistance or as a means to help your body heal and repair itself after some workouts while you focus on staying hydrated.

Whatever your 'why' is, make sure you write it down and keep it close by so that you can quickly remind yourself from time to time.

Setting these objectives will enable you to set certain benchmarks when you need to assess whether or not intermittent fasting 16/8 is working for you or not. You should never fast in order to deprive yourself of food after a binge.

There will be some challenging moments during the day, and your mind needs to be prepared for it so that when they occur, you can overcome them.

Make no mistake about it; intermittent fasting 16/8 – or fasting in general – can be incredibly beneficial, but only if you set about it with the right mindset.

The transition of eating habits

The transition to better and healthier eating habits can be overwhelming, uninspiring, and even paralyzing. This is because you know what you prefer, what you crave, as well as what comforts you. The mere thought that you may have to jettison such foods in order to lead a better life or change your eating habits can be harrowing, emotionally and even physically.

The good news is that eating healthy is not equal to consuming rabbit food. Healthy food can be flavorful and rich and also comes with the bonus of leaving you feeling great and satisfied after the meal.

Here are quick tips that will make your transition to healthier eating simple and straightforward:

- **Do away with junk food**: Remove or do away with unhealthy food in your pantry. No more consumption of chips, pretzels, cookies, microwavable foods, etc. and stock up on fruits, veggies, eggs, nuts, avocado, etc. No one said it is going to be easy, but it is not impossible.
- **Stabilize blood sugars**: When your blood sugar plummets, you will naturally crave sugary and starchy foods. Don't give in to this temptation. Instead, eat vegetables, healthy fats, and proteins.
- **Always shop with a full belly**: Okay, this may not be news, but it must be reiterated. If you go shopping for

groceries on empty stomach, chances are you will submit to the craving to get your blood sugar up. This could push you into making poor food choices.

- **Plan all your meals**: If you do not have a meal plan, you will always succumb to anything that rolls by. And before you blink, you are back right where you started. You can check online meal planning programs if you struggle with meal planning. Choose your meal preferences and your shopping lists and meals will be emailed to you every week.

Most people change their diets because they are tired and sick of feeling sick and tired. But you do not have to wait until you have poor health or in dire need. Be proactive with your health; never take chances that will usher in a crisis.

Remember that there is no medicine like food. Make the right dietary changes, and you will never regret it.

Comfort Foods

Comfort food is food that imparts a sentimental or nostalgic value to someone. It is often characterized by its high carbohydrate level, high caloric nature or simple preparation. The nostalgia, of course, is usually specific to an individual or it may apply to a particular culture.

Comfort foods typically provide a short-term sense of wellbeing, thereby making a person feel good. Foods that are extremely high in sugar, salt or fat elevate the mood by stimulating the reward system in the brain. This is why it is not too uncommon for people to crave French fries, chocolate as well as other foods high in both carbohydrates and sugars.

Many people use comfort food as a means to self-medicate. People with negative emotions usually eat unhealthy foods in an effort to experience and enjoy instant gratification that results in short-lived or temporary good feelings. But then going this route may, in reality, increase the negative feeling instead of quelling them.

A high-carbohydrate-laden meal can cause you to emotionally and physically crash. Most people that consume comfort foods associate them with secure and comforting times or special occasions. The mere smell of comfort foods can entice you to take a bite because there is usually a very strong connection between emotional memory and scent.

When someone overeats, it does much more than activate the reward system. In short, overeating can cause heartburn, upset stomach, nausea, and even vomiting. Both the emotional as well as physical distress that one experiences after eating episodes can be incredibly overwhelming.

There are long-term effects of binge eating, and they include:

- Type 2 diabetes
- Heart disease
- High cholesterol
- High blood pressure
- Depression
- Cancer
- Stroke
- Sleep apnea

The consumption of comfort foods is considered a response to emotional stress and seen as an essential contributor to the epidemic of obesity in the western world. The provocation of specific hormonal responses leads selectively to a sudden increase in abdominal fat.

Further studies have revealed that the consumption of comfort food is triggered by negative emotions in women and by positive ones in men. The stress effect is pronounced explicitly among women of college-age, with only 33 percent reporting very healthy choices during periods of emotional stress.

Examples of comfort foods in the United States include:

- Apple pie
- Burrito
- Beef stew
- Chicken fried steak
- Cake
- Biscuits and gravy
- Chicken soup
- Chili mac
- Chicken and dumplings
- Fried chicken
- Ice cream
- Pizza
- Meatloaf

- Tamale pie
- Grits
- Cupcakes
- Cornbread
- Casseroles
- Pot roast
- Peanut butter
- Green bean casserole
- Tuna casserole, etc.

Examples of comfort foods in Canada include:

- Cheesecakes
- Cookies
- Fried chicken
- Fish and chips
- Fried rice
- Pizza
- Lasagna
- Rhubarb pie
- Scrambled eggs on toast

- Pea soup
- Poutine
- Macaroni and cheese
- Chili and beans, etc.

Examples of comfort foods in the United Kingdom include:

- Cornish pasty
- Custard
- Egg and chips
- Cottage pie (Shepherd's pie)
- Egg and soldiers
- Pies
- Pork pie
- Fish pie
- Steak and kidney pie
- Soups and stews
- Jacket potato
- Bread and butter puddings
- Scotch egg
- Roasted meat, etc.

During intermittent fasting, you may be tempted to consume some comfort foods as a reward for waiting several hours for food. But you should be very careful so that you don't overeat. You should also take care so that you don't end up negating the reason why you fasted in the first place, which is to lose weight and look good.

Chapter Thirteen

Intermittent Fasting 16/8

The simple thought of fasting is often more than enough to make you suddenly hungry. But relax; the benefits of going on an intermittent fasting 16/8. By now, you already the benefits of going on an intermittent fast 16/8.

You can fast in a wide variety of ways, not just total restriction from all foods. At times, fasting may mean avoiding some types of food like fats or even carbohydrates. It may also imply minimizing calories overall.

Intermittent fasting 16/8 helps you to lose weight, improved blood pressure, minimizes risk to cardiovascular diseases, and reduces inflammation, among other things. It can also boost brain function, helps you to live longer, and plays a crucial role in preventing neurodegenerative diseases.

Here are some quick tips to bear in mind before you start your intermittent fast 16/8 journey:

Start Slow

Before your intermittent fasting 16/8, start cutting back gradually on food and drink for several days or even weeks. Or else, beginning an intermittent fasting 16/8 will be a shock for your body.

Don't eat 3 full meals every day with snacks between meals and then abruptly stop eating one day. Your body has become very used to regular refueling, and you may find it somewhat difficult to maintain energy levels during your intermittent fast 16/8.

Therefore, start slow and ease into it before going full throttle.

Eat well

When you engage in an intermittent fasting 16/8, you should endeavor to eat well during your eating window. It is often very tempting to follow up a period of restriction from food by eating a huge meal. But you should fight and overcome that temptation as much as possible.

Breaking your intermittent fasting 16/8 with a feast may leave you feeling tired and bloated. Moreover, if your goal for engaging in an intermittent fast 16/8, feasting may severely harm your long-term goals by considerably slowing down or even halting your weight loss entirely.

Your overall calorie quota significantly impacts your weight. Therefore, if you consume excess calories after a period of restriction from food, it will reduce your calorie deficit.

The best way to break an intermittent fast 16/8 is to continue eating normally – i.e. the same amount you would have had if you were not on a fast – and get back into your regular eating routine.

So, eat enough protein, even if the goal for going on an intermittent fast 16/8 is to try losing excess weight. This is because when you are in a calorie deficit, you will end up losing muscle in addition to excess body fat.

One of the best and quickest ways to minimize or reduce muscle loss while fasting is by ensuring you consume lots of protein during your eating window. Adding a bit more protein to your regular diet when you are on a fast can help to manage your hunger efficiently.

Start Hydrated

It is vital to drink some fluid on an intermittent fasting 16/8. This is because mild dehydration can bring about headaches, fatigue, thirst, and dry mouth. Health authorities often recommend the 8x8 rule, i.e. taking up to eight 8-ounce glasses of fluid every day – which is slightly less than 2 liters in total – in order to stay hydrated.

However, the amount of fluid you need may differ from the amount another person needs. This is because you will often get about 20-30 percent of the fluid that your body needs from eating just food. This is why it is very easy to become dehydrated when engaging in intermittent fasting 16/8.

When fasting, most people consume 8.5-13 cups, i.e. 2-3 liters of clean water over the course of the day. But then, your thirst should tell you whether you need to drink more water or not. Therefore, listen to your body all through the course of the fast.

Avoid Sugary Drinks And Food

Loading up on sweet tea and cookies before undertaking an intermittent fast 16/8 is never a good idea. Of course, you may feel satisfied and full at first, but when your blood sugar drops sharply after an hour or two, you will become extremely hungry and even weak.

Therefore, to have more than enough energy for an extended period, you should only fill up on complex carbohydrates. This includes:

- Carbohydrates, e.g. rice, pasta, and potatoes
- Proteins, e.g. beans, milk, etc.

Sticking to these will give you the energy you need when undertaking an intermittent fast 16/8.

Minimize Intense Activities

It is not often recommended to engage in intense workouts when you are not eating or drinking. This is often the case if you go on a regular fast. However, it was discussed earlier that engaging in workouts while undertaking intermittent fasting 16/8 contributes to weight loss.

Positioning Your Eating Window

Positioning your eating window when engaging in intermittent fasting 16/8 is vital. This is because you don't want to set your fasting hours to periods or hours in which you will be strenuously engaged. Such activities may quickly sap your strength or energy, thereby causing you to break your fast unceremoniously.

Therefore, preserve your energy for vital day-to-day activities since you won't be replenishing your nutrients for the next few hours.

Signs To Watch Out For

During a fast, even an intermittent fast 16/8, it is normal to feel hungry, irritable, and even tired. But you should never feel unwell at all.

If you also become ill or overly concerned about your health, you should stop fasting right away. Some of the signs that you should always watch out for that prevent you from performing your day-to-day tasks include:

- Tiredness

- Weakness
- Discomfort
- Sickness

If you experience these unexpected feelings when undertaking an intermittent fast 16/8, you should stop fasting immediately.

Consider Supplements

If you nearly always engage in intermittent fasting 16/8, you are guaranteed to pass up some essential nutrients. This is because when you reduce your intake of calories, you will find it a bit challenging to meet all your nutritional needs.

It has well been proven that those who follow weight-loss diets are highly likely to be deficient in several essential nutrients such as calcium, vitamin B12, iron, etc.

It is therefore recommended that you consider taking a multivitamin to help prevent these deficiencies as well as for peace of mind. So, do your best to eat whole foods most of the time.

More on supplements will be discussed in the last chapter of this exceptional book.

To wrap up this section, you should know that it is vital to stay healthy while engaging in intermittent fasting 16/8. You can ease into it by starting slow, eating well during the eating window, and staying hydrated as much as possible.

It would help if you also minimized your daily workouts or intense activities, and also take essential supplements in order to replenish your body with the nutrients it needs. Following these will ensure that you maintain optimal health while you enjoy more successful intermittent fast 16/8.

Chapter Fourteen

Metabolism and the Thermic Effect of Food

The thermic effect of food – which is also referred to as postprandial thermogenesis or diet-induced thermogenesis – refers to the increase in metabolic rate, i.e. the rate at which the human body burns off calories. This is an action that occurs right after food intake.

When you eat food, your body is expected to make use of some calories – in the form of energy – to digest, absorb, and then store the nutrients in the food you have ingested. And due to the thermic effect of food, consuming calories enables you to significantly increase the rate via which your body burns off calories.

But then, how does the thermic effect of food affect your metabolic rate? The consensus propounded in the scientific community is that the thermic effect of food accounts for approximately 5-10 percent of the energy content of the food you consume. This implies, for instance, that eating a 400-calorie meal will result in the burning of 20-40 calories in processes like digestion, absorption, and storing of nutrients from the meal. If you eat up to 2,000 calories per day, at least 100-200 calories will be burned every day due to the thermic effect of food.

Fasting is generally equated with starvation. Intermittent fasting 16/8 can be loosely defined in this regard as any fast between twelve and thirty-six hours.

Calorie restriction has been clinically proven to slow down the rate of metabolism. However, short-term fasting with frequent refeeds has the opposite effect.

During an intermittent fast 16/8, the human body is fueled by the burning of fat. And your metabolic rate is increased or maintained by short-term fasting.

A study showed that 8 weeks of intermittent fasting 16/8 significantly reduced fat mass in 34 resistance-trained individuals. Resting metabolic rate (RMR) stayed the same.

Factors Stabilizing Metabolic Rate during Intermittent Fasting
Some factors are known to stabilize the metabolic rate during intermittent fasting.

The metabolic rate – which is also referred to as resting metabolic rate (RMR) or basal metabolic rate (BMR) – is the amount of energy required to power essential bodily functions such as breathing, heartbeat, brainpower as well as other processes that keep you alive and running.

About 60-70 percent of daily expenditure goes towards BMR – though this depends on how physically active you are – while the rest are channeled towards physical activity. If you are very fidgety, you will burn more calories.

Metabolic rate is heavily tied to weight regulation. If your metabolic rate is low, you will burn fewer calories. And the more you will gain weight as you eat X number of calories.

Of course, this analogy is a somewhat simplistic as a carbohydrate calorie has different effects and impacts on the human body than a fat calorie. Moreover, hormones such as insulin, leptin, and a bunch of others have to be accounted for.

In simple words, if the energy in is not equal to the energy out, your weight will show the difference by changing. This is why the concept is known as 'energy balance.'

- **Significant Increase in HGH (Human Growth Hormone):** Intermittent fasting helps to optimize HGH (human growth hormone) in several ways. The eating pattern allows you to shed some body fat which has a direct impact on the production of HGH. This leads to a significant increase of HGH levels which can be up to five-fold (in men) during intermittent fasting. Women, however, do not always experience the same benefits from intermittent fasting that men enjoy. And research is still ongoing to determine whether or not women see the same increase or rise in human growth hormone.

  Asides promoting the burning of fat, HGH also preserve muscle mass along with other benefits.

- **Plummeting Insulin Levels**: Intermittent fasting keeps insulin levels incredibly low for most hours of the day. Insulin levels generally increase whenever you eat. And since you are fasting, there will be no need for the secretion of the hypoglycemic agent.

- **Active Muscle Tissue**: Intermittent fasting, when combined with weight training, engenders the production of functional muscle tissue. This was as a result of fat loss that came about during fat loss caused by intermittent fasting. Getting enough protein during this period is also essential, especially if your aim for undertaking intermittent fasting is to lose excess fat.

Research has made it known that a protein-laden diet can help to preserve muscle during fat loss via intermittent fasting. Protein intakes of approximately 0.7grams/lb of body weight per day (i.e. 1.6 grams/kg) might be sufficient during weight loss. It is highly likely that proper protein intake is particularly vital during intermittent fasting since your body will go for extended periods without receiving any nutrient.

- **Increase in Norepinephrine Hormone Levels**: Norepinephrine is a stress hormone that is actively involved in the 'fight or flight' response. It is known to improve attention and alertness as well as other wide range of effects on the human body. One of such effects of the hormone is informing body cells to release fatty acids.

The increase in norepinephrine hormone levels in the blood typically results in the availability of a substantial amount of fat for the body to burn during intermittent fasting.

All these work together to stabilize the metabolic rate during intermittent fasting.

Chapter Fifteen

Strategic Black Coffee during Intermittent Fasting 16/8

Since intermittent fasting 16/8 began to trend, people are getting used to the concept of not eating for some hours. At least, it has been established that if you eat dinner but skip breakfast the next day so that you can have lunch, you have fasted intermittently. This is simple enough; however, some questions begin to pop up:

- 'Can I have black coffee during my intermittent fasting 16/8?'
- 'What about water? Can I drink water, so I don't become dehydrated?'

Yes, you can have black coffee during your intermittent fasting 16/8 because the beverage has no caloric load. Drinking coffee will not break your fast or sabotage all your weight loss efforts.

When you drink black coffee during an intermittent fast 16/8, you should not add any sweetener like honey, sugar or dairy products like cream and milk. It would help if you avoided any of the numerous delicious treats that many coffee-drinkers usually add to their regular cup of black coffee every morning. This is because most of these treats are loaded with calories that you don't need during the fast.

Although the effect of using these sweeteners is somewhat minimal – i.e. about 100 calories or so – if your primary goal of engaging in intermittent fasting 16/8 is to burn off as much fat as possible, having 100 calories will set you back.

Moreover, intermittent fasting 16/8 teaches you how to overcome habits and practice discipline, even though it is for a limited period.

A cup of regular black coffee, according to the USDA (United States Department of Agriculture), contains less than 5 calories. Even a fluid ounce of black espresso contains approximately 1 calorie. The number of calories present in 1 cup of black coffee is too little to negate the effects or break off intermittent fasting 16/8.

But if you take just 1 ounce of heavy whipping cream – which contains over 100 calories – with a cup of black coffee, you will be ingesting approximately the same number of calories. Take 3 cups of black coffee along with heavy whipped cream, and you will have downed up to 300 calories. This is not an issue if you indulge from time to time. But if it becomes a daily habit, you will find it somewhat challenging to lose or maintain your weight.

Coffee is a very rich and natural source of caffeine which aids weight loss by significantly increasing the rate fat burns in the human body. Thermogenesis or fat burning is the process the human body undergoes when the heat is released via the digestion of the food you take. This helps to speed up metabolism, thereby promoting weight loss.

Caffeine also aids fat or weight loss by drastically reducing appetite. And when appetite is reduced, you will have no need or urge to consume food or excess calories. This is why drinking black coffee has no overall effect on your intermittent fasting 16/8 program asides promoting weight loss.

So, keep drinking that black coffee minus all the sweeteners for as long as possible while you engage in your fast.

Profound Benefits of Black Coffee

Many people love their black coffee first thing in the morning to energize them and get them ready to tackle the issues of the day. But only a handful can answer the question: 'how much do you know about black coffee?' Do you know that drinking coffee affects your body in ways you have never imagined?

Black coffee is coffee that is generally brewed without using any additives like milk, sugar, cream or flavors. It has a more or less bitter taste compared to its flavored variety. But despite this, millions of people around the world love a cup or two of strong black coffee every day. It has become a staple in many people's diets.

Black coffee has the potential to heal if consumed the right way. Drinking black coffee has a plethora of health benefits that many lovers of the beverage are not even aware of. This is because it is overly loaded with nutrients and antioxidants that only a few beverages have.

If you are undertaking intermittent fasting 16/8, you can drink black coffee because it doesn't affect insulin levels. And you can also take caffeinated or decaffeinated coffee during fasting windows. Still, you should not add any milk or sweetener if you don't want to negate the effects of intermittent fasting 16/8. But you can add cinnamon and other related spices to your black coffee. Drinking black coffee supports healthy blood sugar levels over time.

Here are additional benefits of drinking strong black coffee when undergoing intermittent fasting 16/8s:

-Aids In Weight Loss

Black coffee contributes to rapid weight loss, especially if you take a cup of black coffee at least 30 minutes before heading to the gym. It works by making you work out harder in the gym, thereby inducing even more weight loss. This is because adrenaline – or epinephrine – levels in the blood is increased when you take black coffee. This prepares your body and gets it ready for physical exertion. In other words, it works by boosting your metabolism by up to 50 percent, thereby helping you burn belly fat.

Black coffee burns the fat in your tummy since it is a fat-burning beverage. It is known to stimulate the nervous system to break down fat cells, and then use them as a source of fuel or energy – instead of glycogen – during workouts.

-Boosts Cognition

Black coffee contains a considerable amount of caffeine which has been scientifically proven to improve some parts of the human brain that controls concentration and short-term memory. Some research also suggests that caffeine may be linked with a somewhat lower risk of cognitive impairment as well as a lower risk of Alzheimer's disease.

In other words, black coffee boosts brainpower.

-Enhances Liver Health

The human liver is the largest organ in the human body as it conveniently manages more than 500 vital functions almost at the same time. It is very vulnerable to several modern dietary pitfalls, especially if you consume too much fructose or alcohol. It is very important to ensure that it stays healthy at all times.

What many coffee drinkers or lovers don't know is that the liver loves black coffee. Yes, black coffee significantly boosts liver health.

Black coffee helps drinkers to combat diseases like hepatitis, liver cancer, alcoholic cirrhosis, and fatty liver disease. Cirrhosis is considered the end stage of severe liver damage caused by hepatitis and alcoholism. Liver tissues are largely replaced by scar tissue which is not supposed to be.

Multiple in-depth studies have shown that if you take up to 4 cups of black coffee every day, you are among those who are at an extremely low risk of developing liver issues. Drinking the beverage moderately lowers your risk of developing cirrhosis by up to 80 percent. It is also known to lower the risk of liver cancer by up to 40 percent. It also works by reducing the presence of harmful liver enzymes in the blood.

-Antioxidants And Vitamins

Coffee is more than just black water; nearly all the nutrients found in coffee beans successfully make it to the final product. And the final products, i.e. the black coffee you drink, contains decent amounts of minerals and vitamins.

A cup of black coffee contains the following minerals and vitamins:

- 2 percent of the RDA for thiamine (B1) and niacin (B3)
- 3 percent of the RDA for manganese and potassium

- 6 percent of the RDA for vitamin B5 (pantothenic acid)
- 11 percent of the RDA for vitamin B2 (riboflavin)

At first glance, it doesn't look like much, but if you love taking several cups of black coffee per day, it adds up quickly. Black coffee is also loaded with incredible amounts of antioxidants, making it one of the most significant sources of immune-boosting antioxidants found in the modern diet.

A study once reported that roasted coffee beans contain polyphenols, which are the same beneficial and powerful compounds found in red wine, tea, and cocoa. The primary polyphenol in play is chlorogenic acid which is believed to minimize the risk of diabetes and heart disease. This is because chlorogenic acid is loaded with anti-hypertensive, anti-inflammatory, and antioxidant properties, as stated by some Harvard medical specialists. The amount of antioxidants in coffee even outranks many vegetables and fruits.

-Diuretic

Black coffee is a diuretic beverage that makes you urinate as often as possible. Passing out urine as a result of drinking coffee helps to flush bacteria and toxins out easily without any issues. It also helps in cleaning out your stomach.

-Improves the Mood

Drinking several cups of black coffee helps to improve the mood, thereby making you happy. This is possible as caffeine which is present in black coffee, appears to affect the release of the feel-good hormone known as dopamine and serotonin. Dopamine is a neurotransmitter that generates feelings of pleasantness or euphoria, while serotonin is also a neurotransmitter associated with happiness and wellbeing.

Dopamine, which stimulates the specific area of gray matter, is primarily responsible for problem-solving characteristics, alertness, and pressure. These end up making your brain sharper and super active.

This is why the beverage is considered one of the best remedies to fight depression. This conclusion was reached after a meta-analysis of twelve studies involving 346,913 individuals was conducted.

The effects of consuming black coffee which, in turn, generates these feelings of happiness and euphoria, can last well beyond the initial morning mood boost.

So, if you have a bout or two of depression and hope to keep them at bay, take 2 or 3 cups of black coffee every day.

-Minimizes Risk Of Cardiovascular Issues And Diabetes

Harvard researchers have discovered that drinking black coffee minimizes the risk of cardiovascular issues. The caffeine in black coffee constricts the arteries by penetrating the receptors lining the walls of your blood vessels.

This causes your blood pressure to rise appreciably; however, this is a challenge with non-habitual drinkers of black coffee. But this effect on the blood pressure is way smaller in die-hard coffee drinkers. This is because their bodies have become somewhat tolerant to the effect of black coffee. Black coffee also helps to reduce the risk of stroke by up to 22 percent. In other words, black coffee gives you a much healthier heart over time.

Consumption of black coffee also reduces the risk of developing Type 2 Diabetes by up to 7 percent.

What Else Can You Drink During Intermittent Fasting 16/8?

-Water

It has been mentioned in other sections of this book time and again, but it is important to drink water when undergoing intermittent fasting 16/8. Water is – and will always remain – an excellent choice every day, all day long. You can drink sparkling or still water. You can also drink lemon water by squeezing one slice of lemon or lime to your glass of water.

If you love fun flavor variations, consider infusing a pitcher of water with orange slices or cucumber. But stay away from artificially-sweetened water enhancers because it can interfere unfavorably with your fast.

-Tea

If you are looking for that beverage that increases satiety, then tea is your best bet. It is the secret weapon that can make your intermittent fasting 16/8 plan more successful and easier as well.

Green, white, and black teas are synergistic blends of I-theanine and caffeine, which gives drinkers a clean energy boost. This caffeine is different from the variety you get from drinking black coffee. Tea also supports cell health as it contains polyphenols and antioxidants that combat free radicals floating around in your body.

The best types of tea to take when undergoing intermittent fasting 16/8 are:

- Ginger tea
- Green tea
- Hibiscus tea
- Black tea

-Broth

Health specialists highly recommend vegetable broth or bone broth for any period you decide to undergo intermittent fasting 16/8 or a 24-hour fast.

However, you need to beware of bouillon cubes or canned broths. This is because they are often loaded with tons of preservatives and artificial flavors. These additives can considerably counteract the overall effects of your intermittent fasting 16/8.

So, stick to good homemade broths or one that you can obtain from a trusted source.

Incorporating Black Coffee in An Intermittent Fasting Schedule

Incorporating black coffee in your intermittent fasting schedule is not rocket science. As you may have learned by now, you can take black coffee during your intermittent fast. But it must be without sugar, cream, honey or any other sweetener. This will enable you to enjoy the full benefits that the beverage – which also has caffeine – brings to the table.

You can take black coffee early in the morning if that is what you need to keep your mind alert and awake. Bear in mind that you can also take other fluids such as water or 'lemon' water but no sodas or energy drinks.

The goal of taking black coffee is not only to stay alert but to also keep your body hydrated as often as possible. This means that there is no strategic way of taking black coffee since it varies from one person to another.

As long as you black coffee doesn't have any sugar, honey, cream or sweeteners, you can take your beverage at any time of the day, within or outside your eating window.

Chapter Sixteen

Tips Specific to Intermittent Fasting 16/8

The following tips are specific to intermittent fasting 16/8:

Always Check With Your Physician or Healthcare Professional before Engaging in a Fast or a New Diet

Intermittent fasting 16/8 is not for every individual. This includes pregnant or breastfeeding women, and people with type 1 diabetes. Intermittent fasting 16/8 will also not work for those with binge eating disorder. This is because these individuals will overeat during their eating window.

Suppressing Hunger During Intermittent Fasting 16/8

The best ways to suppress hunger as you undertake the intermittent fasting 16/8 method is by:

- **Eating high-fiber foods** such as fruits, vegetables, nuts as well as high-protein foods like tofu, fish, and meat during your eating window. You may also chew high-fiber gummies as it also helps to stave off hunger.

- **Drinking Lots of Water or Black Coffee**: At times, when you think you are hungry, you just may be feeling thirsty. Drink lots of water as well as black coffee without sugar, honey or cream. You can also take licorice herbal teas or cinnamon due to their appetite-suppressing effects.
- **Reduce TV time**: It is easy to 'feel' hungry if you keep seeing ads for food on TV.SS, minimize TV time as much a possible

When to Perform Exercises

It makes no difference one way or the other if you decide to exercise on fasting or feasting ay. However, you may feel a bit more energetic on fasting days if you exercise.

However, you should exercise before you eat since people usually become hungry about 30 minutes after they finish working out. And they may find it very difficult to stick to eating pattern if they can't find something to eat.

But since you are undertaking the intermittent fasting 16/8, you should fast before or during your eating window.

Skipping Breakfast?

Take only black coffee as it helps to boost concentration and energy. It does not have any calories in it as well.

Meditation and mindfulness will go a long way in helping you to feel much better in your fasting period.

Chapter Seventeen

What Are The Four Crucial Healthy Habits Of Life?

If you want to live a long, healthy, happy, and successful life, you need to learn healthy life habits. The pursuit of success has made many individuals take unproven shortcuts with their health, which is detrimental. And before long, they end up suffering one debilitating disease or the other.

It shouldn't be that way at all; no matter how busy you are, you can do a little tweaking in various places in order to develop good habits that will make you live a more productive and healthier life.

Although there are several healthy habits of life, the four most crucial ones are:

1. **Exercise**

If you want to get to the fountain of youth, start a regular exercise regimen. According to the NCI (National Cancer Institute), regular exercise helps maintain healthy bones, joints, and muscles and control weight. It also cuts back the risk of diabetes, high blood pressure, and heart disease.

Exercising your body for 30 minutes, 5-6 days a week is usually recommended by many exercise authorities. You should have one or two days to rest and recuperate. A 30-minute brisk walk can do wonders for your wellbeing or overall health or use a small pedaling device while seated at your desk. So, the exercise doesn't have to be gut-wrenching or anything like that.

2. Nutrition

Eat more nuts and fruits while avoiding snacks and sugary drinks. This is vital to your wellbeing. According to the AHA (American Heart Association), eating a serving of fish (e.g., mackerel, lake trout, sardines, herring, and albacore tuna) at least twice every week will do well for your overall health. This is because these fatty fish are rich sources of omega-3 fatty acids, which significantly reduce the threat and risk of heart disease.

Portion control is also important, so eat larger portions of vegetables and fruits rich in minerals, fiber, and vitamins. Consume small portions of higher-calorie foods with large amounts of fats and sugar.

And don't forget to chew your food. Each mouthful should be chewed 20-30 times in order to get it into its most digestible form. When you chew, it reduces calorie intake by 10 percent, and this is because it takes roughly 20 minutes for your stomach to inform your brain that it is full.

Stop using artificial sweeteners if you want to live up to 100 years. This is because they are associated with diabetes, heart disease, obesity, and long-term weight gain.

3. Whole Foods

The benefits of healthy whole foods cannot be overemphasized. It is the perfect way to get food in its natural state, with all the minerals, vitamins, and other nutrients.

Several extensive studies have shown that a diet rich in healthy foods like whole grains, fruits, and vegetables reduces the risk of diseases like cancer, cardiovascular disease, and type 2 diabetes.

This is because whole foods are loaded with minerals, fiber, and vitamins. They also have phytochemicals i.e., natural compounds in plants. Some of these compounds are antioxidants – such as carotenoids, flavonoids, and lycopene – which protect the cells from damage.

So, stay away from processed foods, which are usually stripped of many healthy nutrients during manufacture. Then they will be added back artificially during the enrichment process. But the final product is often far less nutritious than the whole grains they started with.

4. Stay Hydrated

It is vitally important to get the proper amount of clean water that every tissue, cell, and organ in your body needs. Take at least 8 ounces water every day, though this amount of water has not really been clinically substantiated. A much better guide is to drink enough water that makes you urinate at least once every 2-4 hours. And the urine must have a light color.

You can develop this habit by availing yourself of the numerous free apps and smart bottles on the market today.

Sticking to these four crucial healthy habits of life will not only guarantee sound health but will also prolong your life.

Chapter Eighteen

Sleep

Sleep is highly essential for a person's overall well-being and health, according to the NSF (National Sleep Foundation). It is very much as important as fresh air and food. It is also a vital function that is required to fully support all human lie, development, growth, as well as brain function.

Sleep keeps your mind calm and very alert while assisting you in daily functioning. If you sleep for at least 8 uninterrupted hours and wake up still feeling tired, you do not need more sleep. What you need is a night of better quality sleep. The most important type of sleep your body needs is 'Deep sleep.'

Sleep isn't just a block of time or period when you are not awake or conscious of your surroundings. Sleep studies conducted for several decades has revealed that there are distinct stages of sleep that cycle throughout the night. Forget the myth that your brain is at rest when you are asleep. Your brain remains active throughout the period you are sleeping, even though many different things happen at every stage of sleep.

For instance, in one of the stages of sleep, you feel energetic and well-rested the next day. In another phase of sleep, you make or learn memories.

This implies that during regular nights, people that sleep cycle through several stages. But this begs the question: how much sleep is enough for an individual?

The truth is that sleep needs generally vary from one person to another. These needs change throughout the life-cycle. Most adults, in most cases, need from 7 to 8 hours of sleep every night. Newborns sleep for approximately 16-18 hours a day while kids in preschool may sleep for 10 to 12 hours per day.

However, some individuals have trained their minds and brains to function without drowsiness and sleepiness after only 6 hours of sleep. Other adults cannot perform optimally or at their best unless they have had 10 hours of sleep.

Some people claim that adults do not need too much sleep, especially as they grow older. But there aren't any clinical proofs anywhere to back this belief or claim that older adults can get by with some hours less sleep than younger persons. Older people, however, come awake very quickly at the slightest noise, thereby implying that most of them sleep very lightly.

According to research, six to seven hours sleep is okay for an average individual. The acid test for adequate sleep is whether you are alert or sleep throughout the day. If you are very alert, then it means your sleep is sufficient. But then, sleep is even more important than you probably think right now.

So why is sleep good for you? Does it matter whether or not you get enough sleep?

The answer to both questions is yes, both the quality as well as the quantity of sleep matter a lot. Put differently, how well-rested you are as well as how well you function the following day depends substantially on your total sleep time and how much of the various stages of sleep you get every night.

It is essential for you to always think clearly, react quickly, and also create good memories. The pathways in the human brain that helps us to both learn and remember are incredibly active when we are asleep.

Here are 10 reasons why sleep is super important for a sound and healthy life:

No more confusing thoughts: If you sleep on time, you will no longer have or experience rambling thoughts the next day. This is because the human brain combines recollections when you are resting at night.

No burnouts: If you sleep well for several hours, you will not experience any burnout the next day, especially if the previous day was intellectually and inwardly draining. Getting enough sleep, i.e. 7 to 8 hours of sleep every night, will help you regain anything that may have been depleted in your body due to the activities of the previous day.

Increased risk of stroke, heart disease, etc.: Studies have revealed that poor sleepers are at a high risk of developing heart problems which may result in a stroke. This is why it is crucial to get at least 7 to 8 hours of sleep in order to avoid such risks.

Stay focused: Focus and sleep are proportional to one another. Inadequate sleep leads to lack of focus, and this births many mistakes while completing tasks may take more time.

But when you sleep, you will not be interrupted in any way and this result in complete focus that prompts execution.

Calories: People with disrupted sleep cycles tend to eat more, thereby piling on more calories. And people who get a lot of sleep tend to consume fewer numbers of calories. Sleeping on time allows you to overcome the temptation of snacking at night.

Fat: Many individuals are oblivious of this fact, but lack of sleep considerably leads to the accumulation of fat. Numerous studies have proven that those who do not sleep well are at a very high risk of becoming obese.

Effects of Sleep Deprivation

Depriving yourself of sleep has a price, even though it is often taken lightly. But it is a severe problem as prolonged sleep deprivation can take a severe toll on your health as well as the overall quality of your life.

Sleep deprivation is a pervasive experience that many modern adults face around the world. Most people who strive to make more out of life tend to sacrifice sleep in order to get more work done.

They erroneously believe that less work will result in more productivity. But that is not true, not by a long shot.

Lack of sleep can significantly reduce:

- Productivity
- Effectiveness
- Creativity
- Calmness, etc.

You will do a worse job in whatever you do if you do not sleep well.

Causes of sleep deprivation – aside from the conscious sacrifice of sleep in order to work longer – include:

- Frequent travel
- Stress
- Insomnia
- Shift changes at work
- Blue light from screens like smartphones, laptops, etc.

Insomnia can be caused by the following:

- Depression

- Lack of hormonal balance
- Obstructive sleep apnea, etc.

Sleep deprivation can cause some health problems such as:

- Memory issues
- Trouble with concentration and thinking
- Mood changes
- Accidents
- High blood pressure
- Risk for diabetes
- Weight gain
- Weakened immunity
- Low sex drive
- Poor balance
- Risk of heart disease

Noticeable signs of chronic sleep deprivation include:

- Irritability
- Excessive sleepiness
- Daytime fatigue

- Frequent yawning

Combating Sleep Deprivation

A great place to start is to be aware that you are not getting enough sleep. It is also consequential to understand the harmful effects of sleep deprivation on your overall health and life in general.

However, if you cannot sleep as a result of physical or physiological issues, medical or behavioral treatment may be required.

You can alleviate your deprivation by not exposing yourself to bright lights in the evening, not using your laptop or smartphone in bed, and going to bed on time. Meditation, the use of essential oils, and other medicinal treatments can be used to combat sleep deprivation.

It is often highly recommended that you talk to a physician or healthcare professional if you need to purchase over-the-counter medication in order to combat sleep deprivation.

Exercise

Nearly everyone knows that performing exercises is generally good as it provides profound health benefits. But the modern adult is usually too busy, and despite leading sedentary lifestyles, is too lazy to perform rigorous workouts.

Regular exercise has both short-term and long-term effects on one's overall health. You don't need 5 hours to exercise your entire body; if you can squeeze in 30 minutes of exercise every day, your health will improve drastically.

Breaking the ironclad habit of inactivity is not easy. But if you want to remarkably improve your health, you have no choice than to break free of that sedentary lifestyle that most adults live today and start exercising.

Chapter Nineteen

How to Lose Weight Quickly Without Feeling Frustrated

Losing weight doesn't have to be rocket science. You can lose weight quickly without feeling frustrated. People looking to lose weight tend to get frustrated for the following reasons:

- They look at weight loss as if it is a diet
- They feel deprived, especially when hungry
- They eliminate so-called 'bad foods'

But the truth is you can lose weight without feeling frustrated at all. Here's a quick breakdown of how you can achieve this:

- Avoid fruit juice and sugary drinks
- Always eat a high protein breakfast
- Drink black coffee or tea
- Base your entire diet on whole foods
- Eat only soluble fiber
- Always go for weight-loss friendly foods
- Drinks lots of water before meals which helps in regulating your calorie intake or the amount of food you consume
- Eat slowly, i.e. never eat your meals in a hurry

If you undertake intermittent fasting 16/8 but stick to these tips, that feeling of frustration will ebb off, and you will start seeing some weight loss results.

Benefits of Exercise

Exercise has lots of benefits that you should not hesitate to take advantage of. Here are some of the benefits in no particular order:

- **Improve Your Overall Health**

The benefits obtained from exercise is so profound and numerous that all cannot be listed here. Getting fit minimizes the risk of developing cancer, high blood pressure, diabetes, heart disease, stroke, and so much more.

- **Get More Energy**

Research has shown that performing regular exercises help to minimize tiredness. Exercise itself is an endeavor that is tiring, but one of the ultimate benefits of exercise is that you will eventually feel incredibly energized.

- **Improve Your Mood**

An improved mood is one of the mental benefits of performing exercises. Each time you perform workouts, your body will produce endorphins that help to make you feel good. If you want a natural high, go hard with your exercises!

- **Sleep Better**

It is often easier to have a good night's sleep after undergoing intense exercise. This will eventually add to the energy boost that you obtain from exercise in the long term.

- **Lowers Your Stress Levels**

You can considerably reduce stress levels with exercise. If you have serious mental issues like depression or suffer from stress, regular exercise can greatly minimize the symptoms.

- **Improves Your Appearance**

Exercising to weight loss can provide results. If you are overweight or not toned, you can lose weight to help you feel and look better.

- **Gives You a Sense of Accomplishment**

When you start exercising in order to lose weight and begin to notice improvements every day or each week, you will get a sense of accomplishment that cannot be replicated in any way.

- **Boosts Your Strength and Stamina**

Do you find it a bit challenging to go on long walks even if you want to? Maybe carrying shopping or grocery bags up the stairs leaves you breathless. Go out more; exercise more, and you will eventually be able to handle all these activities without a sweat.

- **Maintain Your Independence Later on in Life**

The more exercise you put in now, the more you can substantially reduce the overall effect of some health problems later in life. Therefore, do your best to keep fit now, and this will help you to remain independent when you are well into the evening of life.

- **Supplements**

The market is full of supplements that are alleged to provide users with healthy weights. You need to be extraordinarily careful, though, as there is no rigid formula to get even one remedy that is devoid of health risks while providing the benefits you crave for.

One of the invaluable supplements you should take from time to time is melatonin. This is the hormone that plays a crucial role in blood pressure and sleep regulation.

Melatonin supplements have become a proven sleep aid that can significantly increase both the duration and quality of your sleep. In order to fully maximize the effect of melatonin supplement, take 1-5mg just 30 minutes before you turn in. You can start with a much lower dose in order to assess your tolerance. Then increase the dose if required.

Although having a good night's sleep – at least 7-8 hours every night – may benefit hormone growth levels, additional research has brought to light the fact that melatonin supplements can directly improve HGH production.

Melatonin is also relatively non-toxic and safe. But then, melatonin may tamper with your brain chemistry in a few ways. This is why you should consider talking to a dietician before purchasing and using weight loss supplements.

Some of the well-known weight loss supplements include:

- Conjugated Linoleic Acid (CLA)
- Chitosan
- Glucomannan
- Ornithine
- L-dopa
- Glutamine
- Glycine
- Creatine

Once again, talk to a dietician before using any weight loss supplement. You may also go online and do your due diligence, read reviews, and watch videos that discuss supplements and their efficacies when it comes to weight loss.

Conclusion

Intermittent fasting 16/8 remains one of the most popular forms of intermittent fasting. The benefits associated with this lifestyle include fat loss, weight loss, as well as the general reduction in the risk of several debilitating diseases such as low blood pressure, diabetes, etc. It has also been proven to combat cancer and helps individuals undergoing chemotherapy treatment.

Intermittent fasting 16/8 is considered in some quarters as a diet plan. But in reality, it is just a lifestyle, an approach to eating that works remarkably well for healthy individuals looking for all the remarkable benefits that fasting has to offer. People that undertake intermittent fasting 16/8 should only focus on eating nutrient-rich, high fiber whole foods and protein-rich diets while ensuring they stay hydrated all through the day.

Take note that intermittent fasting 16/8 is not right for every individual. Anyone who wishes to undertake the intermittent fasting 16/8 method should, first of all, speak to a physician or healthcare professional, especially if they have underlying health conditions or concerns or are on medications.

Intermittent fasting 16/8 should not be embarked on by pregnant women, breastfeeding mothers or those with kidney disease, diabetes, eating disorders as well as any other metabolic disorders. This is because these health conditions can severely alter the human body's storage, balance as well as utilize stores of glucose and insulin, thereby making the intermittent fasting 16/8 method an unsafe or dangerous choice.

More research about intermittent fasting 16/8 is highly required in order to see if and how it can be implemented into a highly effective, weight loss plan.

It is practically impossible for many individuals to restrict food intake entirely for specified periods in order to achieve optimal health. It is difficult socially as no one will likely be happy to skip dinner with friends or boycott happy hours. However, self-imposed rules are understandably not as joyful as possessing the right information that will enable you to make the right choices versus what holds you back.

It is, therefore, in your best interest, to find different ways to make eating nutrient-dense foods work for you as regards your day-to-day life. If you are considering intermittent fasting 16/8, you should give it a try by starting small and working from there all the way up. Keep it as simple as possible. After dinner, close your kitchen and aim to get as much sleep as you can.

So, will you lose weight when you undertake the intermittent fasting 16/8? In theory, yes, you will lose weight. However, it is difficult to really pin down precisely how this type of intermittent fasting will be of enormous benefit to several individuals. This is because the majority of the research carried out on intermittent fasting 16/8 involves people who are overweight or obese and not those who only want to shed off a few pounds. Once again, more research is required to ascertain the overall efficacy of intermittent fasting 16/8 in every healthy individual, obese or not.

Intermittent fasting 16/8 works as long as you undertake it with the primary goal of losing weight since most people overeat at night, and this is a factor that contributes significantly to weight gain. Fasting will do away with that unpleasant obstacle. Of course, the timing of your eating window can considerably impact how much weight you shed off over time.

Undertake the intermittent fasting 16/8 with a positive mindset, don't binge on snacks or consume junk food during your 8-hour eating window, and be as consistent as possible. If you love midnight snacks, this is the time to scrap those inhibiting and informal meals throughout the specified period of your fasting.

Do not expect a sudden and miraculous slim-down to happen overnight. Set your mind for the 16 hangry hours ahead as soon as you embark on the program. And be willing to push through it all, come hell or high water.

Printed in Great Britain
by Amazon